TRANS AND GENDER DIVERSE AGEING IN CARE CONTEXTS

Research into Practice

Edited by
Michael Toze, Paul Willis and Trish Hafford-Letchfield

With forewords by
Shanna K. Kattari and Pauline Smith

First published in Great Britain in 2024 by

Policy Press, an imprint of
Bristol University Press
University of Bristol
1–9 Old Park Hill
Bristol
BS2 8BB
UK
t: +44 (0)117 374 6645
e: bup-info@bristol.ac.uk

Details of international sales and distribution partners are available at policy.bristoluniversitypress.co.uk

© Bristol University Press 2024

British Library Cataloguing in Publication Data
A catalogue record for this book is available from the British Library

ISBN 978-1-4473-7001-7 hardcover
ISBN 978-1-4473-7002-4 paperback
ISBN 978-1-4473-7003-1 ePub
ISBN 978-1-4473-7004-8 ePdf

The right of Michael Toze, Paul Willis and Trish Hafford-Letchfield to be identified as editors of this work has been asserted by them in accordance with the Copyright, Designs and Patents Act 1988.

All rights reserved: no part of this publication may be reproduced, stored in a retrieval system, or transmitted in any form or by any means, electronic, mechanical, photocopying, recording, or otherwise without the prior permission of Bristol University Press.

Every reasonable effort has been made to obtain permission to reproduce copyrighted material. If, however, anyone knows of an oversight, please contact the publisher.

The statements and opinions contained within this publication are solely those of the editors and contributors and not of the University of Bristol or Bristol University Press. The University of Bristol and Bristol University Press disclaim responsibility for any injury to persons or property resulting from any material published in this publication.

Bristol University Press and Policy Press work to counter discrimination on grounds of gender, race, disability, age and sexuality.

Cover design: Robin Hawes
Front cover image: istock/nito100

Trish dedicates this to her grandchildren Nora and Teddy, the new gen(d)eration.

Thanks to all those older people and allies who have shared their insights, knowledge and skills with us – we are still and always listening and learning.

Contents

List of figures and tables	vii
Notes on contributors	viii
Acknowledgements	xiii
Foreword	xiv
Shanna K. Kattari	
Foreword: Trans ageing	xvi
Pauline Smith	
Introduction: Trans ageing and care – a review of the terrain	1
Michael Toze, Paul Willis and Trish Hafford-Letchfield	

PART I What do we know about older trans people's lives and care needs? Messages from research

1	Trans and gender diverse ageing and the life course: what can evidence from quantitative studies tell us about how trans people age?	15
	Dylan Kneale, Evangeline Tabor and Laia Bécares	
2	"I need to get on with it": experiences of older trans people navigating healthcare	41
	Evelyn Callahan, Ben Vincent and Richard Holti	

Over to you	55

PART II Perspectives from practice: views, attitudes and practices of healthcare and welfare professionals

3	"You know what? I'm not agreeing": older trans people's experiences of navigating, building and refusing care	61
	Michael Toze	
4	Not in the family: trans people's experiences of family relationships and the implications for support in later life	77
	Trish Hafford-Letchfield, Christine Cocker, Keira McCormack and Rebecca Manning	
5	"What happened to my body over the past decade?" Trans masculine ageing and embodiment in a cisgenderist and ageist society	91
	Alexandre Baril	
6	Examining the views and attitudes of health and social care professionals towards older trans people: findings from the Trans Ageing and Care study	107
	Deborah Morgan, Paul Willis and Christine Dobbs	

7	Professional preparedness for supporting older transgender adults when working in social services in Sweden *Sofia Smolle*	120
8	Gender-affirming surgery in later life: centring older adults' perspectives to promote equitable access and person-centred surgical care *Elijah R. Castle and Laura L. Kimberly*	134
9	What is being done to support trans older people facing intimate and domestic abuse? *Trish Hafford-Letchfield and Keira McCormack*	152

Over to you 173

PART III Making care practices more inclusive: perspectives on improving care and support for trans people in later life

10	Trans history as cultural competence *Kit Heyam*	179
11	Reframing gender neutrality in dementia care cultures *Phil Harper*	190
12	End-of-life care needs and considerations for older trans people *Kathryn Almack, Olivia Warnes and Eloise Kane*	204

Over to you 215

Conclusion: Looking ahead for enabling trans-inclusive and affirming practice 221
Paul Willis, Michael Toze and Trish Hafford-Letchfield

Index 226

List of figures and tables

Figures
1.1	Distribution of gender identities among older trans people aged 55+ in England and Wales	23
1.2	Distribution of gender identities among quantitative studies of older trans lives and ageing	29
8.1	Recommendations to improve the state of gender-affirming surgical care for older trans adults	143

Tables
1.1	Overview of included study characteristics	25
6.1	Statements assessing respondents' knowledge of key legal and medical requirements	113
9.1	SafeLives DASH LGBTQ+ questions	164

Notes on contributors

Kathryn Almack (she/her) is Professor of Family Lives and Care (School of Health and Social Work, University of Hertfordshire) and Honorary Professor of Inclusive Health and Social Care at the University of Nottingham. Kathryn is a sociologist, and her research addresses relationships of care in people's lives. This includes a substantial focus on lesbian, gay, bisexual and trans (LGBT+) older people's experiences of ageing and end-of-life care. She has published widely in this area and has an effective sustained track record of her research being used to shape and influence policy and professional practice. ORCID ID: 0000-0002-4342-241X

Alexandre Baril (he/him) is Associate Professor at the University of Ottawa. His work is situated at the crossroads of gender, queer, trans, disability/crip/Mad studies, critical gerontology and critical suicidology. His commitment to equity has earned him awards for his involvement in queer, trans and disabled communities, including the Canadian Disability Studies Association Tanis Doe Francophone Award (2020) and the Equity, Diversity and Inclusion President's Award at the University of Ottawa (2021). A prolific author, he has given over 200 presentations and has 80 publications. He is the author of *Undoing Suicidism: A Trans, Queer, Crip Approach to Rethinking (Assisted) Suicide* (2023). ORCID ID: 0000-0003-4833-1979

Laia Bécares (she/her) is Professor of Social Science and Health at King's College London. Her work examines the mechanisms by which structural oppression, including heterosexism and cisgenderism, leads to health and social inequities over the life course. ORCID ID: 0000-0002-4207-074X

Evelyn Callahan (they/them) is a research fellow at University College London working with older people living in almshouses. Their other research interests include trans healthcare, healthcare in resource-limited settings and applied qualitative research methods. They have a PhD in sociology from Brunel University London, an MSc in medical anthropology from University College London and a BA in anthropology from the University of Connecticut. ORCID-ID: 0000-0002-0360-4657

Elijah R. Castle (he/him) is a study coordinator with the Hunter Alliance for Research and Translation, working on projects related to trauma-informed approaches to healthcare and research, sexual health for trans men and trans masculine people, health education and knowledge dissemination and community engagement. For over five years, Elijah has provided peer and community support and education on topics related to trans healthcare and surgery navigation (especially genital surgeries). He has also worked in gender-affirming surgery research and medical case management. He is particularly interested in research related to patient–provider relationships as well as the relationship between trans surgeries and embodiment. ORCID ID: 0000-0003-0894-2214

Christine Cocker (she/her) is Professor in Social Work and Head of School at the University of East Anglia, Norwich, UK, and a qualified social worker. Prior to academia, Christine practised in child and family social work. She continues to have strong links with practice as an independent member of a Local Authority Fostering Permanence Panel and as Independent Chair for a Local Authority's Children's Academy and as an author of Safeguarding Adult Reviews. Her research and publications are in the area of social work with looked-after children, LGBT+ issues in social work and transitional safeguarding. ORCID ID: 0000-0002-4188-2316

Christine Dobbs (she/her) is based at the Centre for Innovative Ageing, Swansea University. As a Chartered Psychologist, joined the Centre for Innovative Ageing after completing her PhD in 2008 and worked here almost continuously until taking on her current position as Honorary Research Fellow in December 2020. Prior to this, she was Postgraduate Programme Director for Gerontology and Ageing Studies. She has held a number of roles in research, teaching and student supervision. Research has included end-of-life care for older people, as well as intra- and intergenerational relationships in black and minority ethnic elders elders, and, more recently, looking at dignified and inclusive health and social care for older trans people living in Wales. ORCID ID: 0000-0002-4320-6709

Trish Hafford-Letchfield (she/her) is Professor of Social Work at the University of Strathclyde, Scotland, UK. She is a qualified nurse and social worker. Her research interests are in the experiences of ageing of people in marginalised communities, and much of her research uses participatory methods. She has published extensively on LGBTQ+ ageing and care; on suicide thought and behaviour and problematic substance use in later life; educational gerontology; leadership and management; and organisational development in social work and social care. Trish has over 150 publications including 20 books which more recently have included *Rethinking Feminist Theories for Social Work Practice* for Palgrave with Christine Cocker, and she is also series and volume editor on the series on Sex and Intimacy in Later Life with Paul Simpson and Paul Reynolds for Policy Press. Orchid ID: 0000-0003-0105-0678

Phil Harper (they/them) is Senior Lecturer in Health and Social Care at Birmingham Newman University. Phil is currently studying for a doctorate, where they aim to explore care staff's understanding of the needs of non-binary individuals living with dementia. Phil has also been involved in research projects looking at transgender individuals' experiences of healthcare and personal care for people living with dementia. Phil is also an advisor/LGBTQ+ consultant for the Association for Dementia Studies and external member of the Northampton Dementia Research Centre. Phil is also part of Alzheimer's Europe's working group on Sexuality and Gender, where they helped to develop resources around LGBTQ+ inclusion in policy and practice. Phil is currently Chair of the conference subgroup in the LGBTQ+ Dementia Advisory group. ORCID ID: 0000-0003-0933-005X

Kit Heyam (they/he) is a writer, researcher, heritage practitioner and trans awareness trainer who has supported a wide variety of professionals across the UK to develop trans inclusivity. Their research investigates the history of gender and sexual non-conformity, and their 2022 book *Before We Were Trans: A New History of Gender* – which argues for the importance of understanding gender-non-conforming people on their own historical and cultural terms – was a finalist for the 2023 Lambda Literary Award in Transgender Nonfiction. They are currently working with the Royal Armouries Museum and University of Plymouth to illuminate gendered aspects of the museum's collection. ORCID ID: 0000-0001-7541-7001

Richard Holti (he/him) is Professor of Professional Learning at the Open University. He recently led the research team funded by the UK National Institute for Health and Care Research on the project 'Improving the integration of care for trans adults' (ICTA). Learning also from the experiences of his trans son, he is committed to improving the healthcare that trans people receive. ORCID ID: 0000-0003-4769-8621

Eloise Kane (she/her) is Consultant in Palliative Medicine, Marie Curie Hospice Bradford, caring for patients with life-limiting illness. She has a passion for inequalities work including developing local services for prisoners, chairing her local palliative care network's equity, diversity and inclusion committee. She has a particular focus on LGBTQ+ communities, especially the trans community, and provides education sessions on this topic. She was also involved in supporting the Hospice UK 'I just want to be me' report in 2023. ORCID ID: 0000-0003-3241-6054

Laura L. Kimberly (she/her) is Assistant Professor in the Hansjörg Wyss Department of Plastic Surgery and in the Division of Medical Ethics in the Department of Population Health at New York University Grossman School of Medicine in New York City, USA. Her research examines ethical and psychosocial considerations in innovative surgical interventions, including gender-affirming surgery. Her work seeks to centre patients' lived experiences of embodied identity over the life course. ORCID ID: 0000-0001-6873-6266

Dylan Kneale (he/him) is a principal research fellow at the EPPI-Centre, UCL Social Research Institute, University College London. He is particularly interested in ageing, LGBTQ+ health, social exclusion and evidence-informed decision making, as well methods involving evidence synthesis and secondary data analysis. ORCID ID: 0000-0002-7016-978X

Rebecca Manning (she/her) is a registered mental health nurse and manager of a community mental health team in Suffolk at the Norfolk and Suffolk Foundation NHS Trust and has experience in the gender field, through personal experience, founding and running a social enterprise to support the trans community and working with people in both the health and charity sectors, and was recently part of the Clinical Reference Group for NHS England. ORCID ID: 0000-0003-0076-9103

Keira McCormack (she/they) is a senior independent domestic violence advisor (IDVA), having working intensely within both the domestic abuse and sexual abuse fields and previously spending 15 years as a counsellor in rape crisis settings. Keira set up and ran a counselling charity in Belfast aimed at the trans, non-binary and intersex community. She is also on the board of an LGBT charity in Belfast, Northern Ireland. ORCID ID: 0009-0002-8509-6904

Deborah Morgan (she/her) is a senior research officer in the Centre for Innovative Ageing, Swansea University. Her main research interests are loneliness and social isolation in later life and she has a PhD. She sits on the Welsh government Loneliness and Social Isolation Strategy Board and is a member of the Cross Party Intergenerational Solidarity Group. Deborah's research has led to several invited national and international presentations, and she has made several appearances on radio and television. She is also a TEDx Swansea speaker. ORCID ID: 0000-0002-3107-3945

Sofia Smolle (they/them) is a PhD student in social work at the Department of Psychology and Social Work at Mid Sweden University. Areas of interest are transgender and queer perspectives including queer ageing, intersectionality, norm-critical approaches, empowerment, social welfare, knowledge-enhancing initiatives regarding critical and radical social work and LGBTQ+-related activism. ORCID ID: 0000-0003-0960-8832

Evangeline Tabor (they/them) is a final-year PhD candidate at University College London funded through the Soc-B CDT (ESRC/BBSRC). Their work examines LGBTQ+ health disparities and inequities across the life course. Their current interests include queer data ethics, the measurement of sexuality in large population surveys, LGBTQ+ physical health inequities, LGBTQ+ ageing and queer joy. ORCID ID: 0000-0002-5485-8817

Michael Toze (he/him) is Senior Lecturer in Public Health and Social Determinants of Health at Lincoln Medical School, UK. Prior to academia, Michael worked in local government policy. Michael has been involved in running trans masculine support groups for over 15 years and has published on topics relating to trans health, ageing and LGBT+ communities. ORCID ID: 0000-0003-4699-9190

Ben Vincent (they/them) is an independent scholar and author of the books *Transgender Health* (2018) and *Non-binary Genders* (2020). They are a co-editor of the collections *Non-binary Lives* (2020) and *TERF Wars* (2020). Ben was also a co-author of the eighth edition of the WPATH Standards of Care and recently worked as Research Coordinator of the Trans Learning Partnership, based at the charity Spectra. ORCID ID: 0000-0002-3110-3008

Olivia Warnes (she/her) is Policy and Advocacy Officer at Hospice UK. Following a masters in global governance, Olivia joined Hospice UK in 2021. Since then, she has worked closely with Gender Identity Research and Education Society (GIRES)and Stonewall on a programme of work examining trans and gender diverse communities' access to and experiences of palliative and end-of-life care, resulting in the publication of the 2023 report 'I just want to be me'. Olivia has a longstanding interest in human rights and health inequalities. Her work in the trans healthcare space continues with further research and advocacy projects. ORCID ID: 0009-0004-5072-6536

Paul Willis (he/him) (PhD) is Professor of Social Care in the School of Social Sciences, Cardiff University, and a registered social worker. His research areas include: older men's experiences of loneliness and social isolation; sexuality, care and ageing; trans ageing and gender identity; inclusive housing and care provision for diverse groups of older people; and social work practice with older people. Paul has a longstanding interest in the ageing experiences of people from sexual and gender minoritised groups. He has recently co-edited a new international volume entitled *Ageing, Men and Social Relations* (2023) (published by Policy Press as part of their Ageing in a Global Context series). ORCID ID: 0000-0002-9774-0130

Acknowledgements

Thanks to SafeLives for their kind permission to reproduce the DASH checklist in Chapter 9. This checklist was developed and published by SafeLives and can be freely downloaded from: https://safelives.org.uk/sites/default/files/resources/Dash%20without%20guidance.pdf. SafeLives are a UK registered charity (no 1106864).

Foreword

Shanna K. Kattari

As someone who has been working in LGBTQIA+ activism for over two decades, I can speak about how often older adults are left out of these spaces. Whether for activism, social engagement, health or other facets of life, LGBTQIA+ spaces tend to centre around young people and sometimes middle-age individuals, leaving out older adults, to the detriment of the community at large. I embarked on a video project, funded by the Rose Community Foundation, entitled 'Protecting Our past: LGBTQ Jews and social justice', with the express purpose of interviewing LGBTQ Jewish elders to ensure their wisdom and experiences were not lost. It was an incredibly engaging and heart-warming experience to listen to their stories of running underground lesbian switch boards to connect one another and marching with Martin Luther King Jr in Alabama, because all of our liberation is tied together.

However, while the field of gerontology has grown exponentially, and research on and with trans communities has exploded in the past few years, there is still an incredible dearth of information on the experiences of transgender older adults, and there is even less available research on older adults who are gender diverse. Most of the extant work speaks only to trans and gender diverse elders going back into the closet or detransitioning for safety as they go into communal living spaces or explores all of the incredibly terrifying rates of discrimination, harassment and victimisation that this group faces in healthcare settings. *Trans and Gender Diverse Ageing in Care Contexts: Research into Practice* serves to bridge some of these gaps by inviting a plethora of authors from around the world to share their research findings and practice experiences in supporting trans and gender diverse older adults in a variety of care contexts. Importantly, this book features many authors who are themselves older adults, trans and/or gender diverse, or both, centring the voices of this community rather than speaking over or for them.

From centring the need for providers and community members to more intimately understand trans history and its impact on trans and gender diverse older adults in today's society to sharing what trans and gender diverse older adults have to say about surgery, hormones, aging bodies and end-of-life care, Michael Toze, Paul Willis and Trish Hafford-Letchfield have created a wonderful resource for social service and healthcare providers alike to truly understand many of the nuanced needs facing those at the intersection of a marginalised gender and aging. Whether you opt to read this from cover to cover in a linear fashion or start where you are most interested and go from there, I am delighted that this book exists and hope that it sparks more international conversations on how we can better support trans and gender diverse people as they age, in all contexts. Our trans and gender elders, soon to be our 'transcestors', are a deeply valuable part of our community and deserve to be heard, upheld and supported in the same way that they have done in leading the way for the rest of us.

In solidarity,
Shanna K. Kattari

Foreword: Trans ageing

Pauline Smith

Being transgender is never easy, yet it's not a curse but a gift. None of us choose to be trans; it's who we are. Like many of us, I knew at an early age that I was in the wrong body – I couldn't change it at nine or in the decades since. It was a secret I hid from family and friends, only dressing alone in private as a girl and then a woman.

At almost 50, I came out in Holland as Pauline and had two years of therapy to find out why I am different, and I learned to love myself and to build my self-esteem ... *zelfvertrouwen* in Dutch, which encompasses self-esteem and self-love.

Life was not magically simpler, but accepting myself and loving myself made it more worthwhile, and I learnt to be an advocate for the trans community and to fight for us to be treated with respect and dignity as ordinary people.

This book is about how we want to be treated as we age – whether it's being looked after in our homes, in hospitals, in care homes or hospices. All we ask is that you treat us with respect and dignity; as we age, we will make mistakes and sometimes appear to be the gender we were born as rather than the one we have chosen.

Many of us are estranged from our blood family, and our friends have become our family unit now. Please do not misgender us, and show us compassion and accept that our family unit is not always conventional.

There are many words of wisdom in this research; please read it and listen to why it's important for all who are transgender like me.

It means a lot to me and all of us who contributed to this research. We are really just ordinary people, your sister or brother, grandad or grandma, aunt or uncle or your parent ... or neighbour.

Treat us as you would them: with kindness and respect.

This is a poem I have written for this book about what it's like being transgender as an older person and what I hope will happen after you read this book.

Being Transgender and ageing

It's hard being who we are
That special gift
To be both genders
And understand
The differences and similarities

Foreword: Trans ageing

And as we age we look
For acceptance, tolerance
Understanding and empathy
It's not much to ask for … we truly hope

Many of my peers came out
Later in life
Frightened of daring to take that huge step
And be vilified and abused
Discrimination it's called

I'm 75 now, trans and proud of who I am
Comfy as me in my own skin
Being Pauline is me
But I worry about my declining years

What will happen to me
In hospital, a care home, a hospice
Will I be able to be safe
Will the nurses and carers treat me
And give me care as who I am
Or who they see

Can I still be Pauline
Needing a shave and wanting
To wear my nightie
Or will they say
You are a man

Let me and my peers
Retain our dignity
Respect our wants and treat us
As we want to be treated

And learn from the words in this book

                                              Thank you,
                                             Pauline Smith

Introduction: Trans ageing and care – a review of the terrain

Michael Toze, Paul Willis and Trish Hafford-Letchfield

Introduction

There has been growing attention to the needs of trans, non-binary and gender diverse populations from the 2010s onwards. Political and media discussion of the issue has often been heated and has tended to associate gender diversity with youth, sometimes presenting this as a generational 'divide'. While there certainly has been a rise in the number of younger people openly expressing and exploring different identities, gender diversity is not a new phenomenon. Older gender diverse people are already accessing ageing services, and younger generations will need such services as they age. As the ageing population continues to grow, so will the number of gender diverse people seeking additional housing, welfare, health and social care and community-based support in later life. Professionals and practitioners who work with older people therefore need to be aware of the potential needs of gender diverse service users and consider how to make their services more inclusive. In 2023, the World Health Organization (2023) announced plans to develop guidelines on improving access and quality of care for trans and gender diverse people, in response to perceived need.

This book aims to support practitioners by exploring the context of gender diversity in ageing and providing practical guidance for practitioners who work with older people in a range of settings. In this introduction, we provide an overview of key terminology and concepts relevant to this subject area, which are then developed in more depth in three main sections. Part I explores what we know about older trans and gender diverse people from existing research. Part II explores perspectives from practice in a range of health, wellbeing and care settings. Part III considers how services can be made more inclusive, with a focus on identifying barriers and considering alternative perspectives on inclusivity. Each section incorporates activities and reflections to help you apply the information to your own professional or academic context. We have labelled these activities as 'Over to you' to reflect a focus on self-directed learning and application to your own practice.

Terminology

Key terms used within this book include trans, non-binary and gender diversity. **Trans** is a broad term, generally understood to encompass anyone who does not feel comfortable with the gender assigned at birth and/or with the gendered categories they continue to be assigned by society and the state (Pearce, 2018b). Many trans people consider themselves to be men or women and use trans as an adjective to these terms, so **trans man** or **trans woman** in line with the individual's current gender identity. **Non-binary** people do not identify as being a man or a woman. They may consider themselves to have no gender, a gender that is something other than male or female, a gender that encompasses both male and female aspects and/or a fluid sense of gender (Vincent, 2018). Many non-binary people consider themselves to be trans, but others may not.

Cis or **cisgender** are antonym terms to trans, used to refer to individuals who do still broadly identify with the gendered categories assigned to them at birth. (In Latin, 'trans' means to go across, whereas 'cis' means to stay on the same side.) Terms such as **cisnormative** and **cisgenderism** relate to social expectations that treat being cisgender as the norm and discriminate against people who are not cisgender. Ansara (2012, 2015) defines cisgenderism as a pervasive ideology in which individuals self-defining their gender are perceived as inferior or invalid in comparison to cisgender people. Cisgenderism is expressed across several levels: individual (for example, misgendering a person, refusing to recognise someone as trans/ by their stated gender); structural (for example, introducing or tightening legal requirements that trans individuals must meet in order to be recognised by their gender); and institutional (for example, where state-recognised legitimacy of an individual's gender identity is subject to medical scrutiny and approval) (Ansara, 2012). In a similar vein, cisnormative discourse perpetuates a taken-for-granted assumption that all people are cisgender and will remain so throughout the life course (Bauer et al, 2009). This is the normative standpoint by which trans lives are judged by and consequently positioned as deviant or disruptive.

However, the desire to present neat definitions can elide wider issues. 'Trans' is an umbrella term intended to group together people aligned with earlier descriptions such as transvestite, transsexual and transgender (Pearce, 2018b). Many of these earlier terms originated within European and North American sexological research and were later incorporated in diagnostic classifications. This medicalised history means that individual and community relationships with these terms are complex and contested. Some people may strongly identify with medical categories, to the extent of rejecting 'trans' because it loses that specificity. Others perceive medical terminology as pathologising, or simply see medical perspectives as less relevant to their experiences. More recent medical texts have sought to draw back from this debate, stating that gender diversity is not in itself a medical issue and seeking to distinguish between diagnostic terms and community identities (American Psychiatric Association, 2013). Nonetheless, regardless of the intention of presenting 'trans' as an umbrella term that moves away from medical history, not everyone who could be covered by the broad definition of trans necessarily feels included. Equally, evolving understandings of what it is to be trans may also bring into question what it is to be cis and whether it is necessarily helpful to present trans/cis as a new binary.

One area of concern is the extent to which Western perspectives on gender, Anglophone terminology and the history of medicalised diagnosis may be crowding out other accounts and experiences of gender diversity. Populations such as *hijra* in India, *fa'afafine* in Samoa, Two Spirit in some North American indigenous communities or *travesti* in Latin America certainly fall outside the male/female binary, but attempting to envelope them under the Anglophone term and concept of 'trans' elides important differences in experiences, cultural location and issues (Towle and Morgan, 2006; Mount, 2020). Towle and Morgan (2006) highlight how there can also be elements of exoticisation or romanticisation in such discussions, extracting culturally specific experiences and concepts to support narratives that suit the Global North rather than centring the concerns and needs of those populations. Choice of terminology around gender identity may also directly intersect with other social divisions such as class and ethnicity and can both reinforce and challenge other normative social structures around gender (Valentine, 2007; Mount, 2020). Balanced against these debates about the nature of gender may be issues of strategic and political activism: while medicalisation of trans identities is subject to justifiable critique, medicalised narratives may also at times be pragmatically useful in securing individual access to gender-affirming interventions and collective access to legal protections. As a consequence of these debates and contentions around the word 'trans', the term **gender diversity** is also used to include other forms of identities or experiences outside the expected norms of male or female.

Within a book on ageing, it is also important to note generational divides on terminology and identity. Terms that are familiar and comfortable to one generation may be rejected as out of date or conceptually problematic by the next. Lists of inclusive terminology may tend to represent the preferences of those who are currently most active in trans-specific groups and spaces, which may in turn tend to be biased towards younger adults. For instance, since the start of the 21st century, the tendency in the Global North has been for 'transsexual' to be replaced by 'transgender', and for that to then be replaced by terms such as 'trans man' or 'trans woman', to the extent that the term 'transsexual' may now be seen as outdated or even offensive (Ram et al, 2022; Thelwall et al, 2022). However, older community members may not necessarily see the need to change their self-descriptors to meet the preferences of following generations.

It is common for trans people to change their names, titles and pronouns (for example, 'he', 'she', 'they' or neo-pronouns like 'zie'). For some, this will occur alongside a permanent change in their gender presentation, often called social **transition**. Transition often but not always also includes legal and/or medical processes, for example seeking legal recognition of gender change through amending documents such as birth certificates and/or seeking gender-affirming medical care. Trans people making this kind of permanent transition will often want all documents and records to correctly reflect their new identity and may not wish to have their trans status revealed without their consent. Other trans people may decide not to make changes to their names, titles and pronouns, or their usage may be fluid or contextual. For instance, they may have changed their name within social settings but not at their place of employment, or they may sometimes use a more masculine name and sometimes a more feminine one.

Some trans people may not be able to make their preferred changes to their individual personal details, particularly on formal documents such as identification or health records. Sometimes this may be temporary, for example because they are awaiting the conclusion of a legal or administrative process to formally change their details. In other cases, it may be impossible for the individual to receive recognition in the way they would want, for example because they are non-binary but the state only permits male and female categories. There may be non-statutory processes that nonetheless create a barrier, such as healthcare systems that require recorded gender to match insurance details and/or the type of care being received, making it difficult for a trans man to access gynaecological care while recorded as male. There are also countries in which gender diversity is illegal or subject to persecution, where documenting any details at all may place individuals at risk. One attempt to map the criminalisation of gender diversity can be viewed on the Human Dignity Trust (2023) website. While professionals should be as flexible as possible in affirming the identities of people using their services, it is also necessary to consider the local context and be alert to the possibility that in some cases there may be other risks and harms to consider. Any such challenges should be discussed with the client concerned to try to reach the most appropriate solution.

In summary, therefore, terminology, categories and underlying concepts around trans and non-binary identity and gender diversity are contextual, historically situated and frequently changing. Any specific advice offered here may not be appropriate in all countries and contexts and may quickly go out of date. Our advice on terminology is to listen to the people you work with, their significant others and their communities and reflect back the terminology they prefer. On an individual level, this requires respecting personal choices around name, title, pronoun and other descriptors. It is important to be aware that there may be different perspectives on terminology within communities, and these may intersect with other social considerations such as race, age and class. In the context of supporting older people, the intersection between age, ageism and gender identity is highly pertinent to this volume, and several authors in this book elaborate on the social and cultural impacts of these intersections. In Chapter 1, Kneale et al explore the quantitative evidence on older trans lives and highlight some of the challenges in exploring varied self-descriptors and life trajectories within standardised datasets. In Chapter 10, Heyam considers the dynamic and historically contingent nature of trans identity. And in Chapter 5, Baril undertakes an autoethnographic exploration of ageing and change in the context of cisnormativity.

The demographics of trans, non-binary and gender diverse ageing

Complexities around terminology also generate difficulties in trying to map trans, non-binary and gender diverse ageing. Until well into the 21st century, demographic measures such as censuses, health service records and population surveys typically did not collect data on gender diverse populations. While wider data collection has been attempted in recent years, as discussed in more detail in Chapter 1, there remain practical and conceptual difficulties in asking questions about gender identity that recognise diversity within the population while also being comprehensible and acceptable to all (Lyons et al, 2021; Schilt and Bratter, 2015). In addition, many within trans communities have justifiable concerns about how their data will be used by governments, public bodies and academia and hence may opt not to disclose their trans status, no matter how well worded the question (Meier and Labuski, 2013).

As a consequence, we do not yet have full clarity on the demographics of gender diverse populations. It is likely that existing data tend to both underestimate the size of the population and underrepresent certain groups within the populations. Historically, data collection primarily focused upon those making a permanent medical transition, and even today it may be easier to measure populations who have taken specific steps such as receiving a medical diagnosis or making a legal name change (Meier and Labuski, 2013; Goodman et al, 2019). It is plausible that those who experience economic precarity, discrimination or intersecting marginalisations may be most concerned about the implications of disclosing their trans status and hence be less likely to do so. As such, any discussion of the needs of older gender diverse populations probably underrepresents the concerns and challenged faced by those in the Global South, those who are not in contact with formal services and those who are subject to multiple marginalisations, among others.

Another empirical challenge is the often hidden nature of trans lives and experiences in LGBT research studies where findings specific to trans older people are conflated with those of older LGB adults across samples (Witten, 2014a; Waling et al, 2019). This can lead to a form of 'coercive queering' in which trans individuals are assumed to be LGB (Ansara, 2015) and highlights the importance of focusing on trans adults' health and wellbeing separately from issues pertinent to sexual orientation and sexual minority groups (while recognising that many trans people will identify as LGB and/or queer and experience similar forms of marginalisation encountered by others in these groups).

Data consistently report that older populations are less likely to identify themselves as trans, non-binary or gender diverse compared to younger ones (Goodman et al, 2019; Office for National Statistics, 2023). This generational change may reflect a number of factors. In part, it may relate to some of the terminological issues mentioned earlier: perhaps we are not asking older people about their gender in the right way. However, it is also likely that the growing numbers of younger people coming out as trans, and the comparatively small number of older people doing so, is linked to the legal and social barriers that existed in the past and the difficulties older people may have faced in exploring their identities and finding supportive communities across the life course.

Gender diversity and the life course

Witten (2009) suggests three potential life trajectories for trans older people: (i) those who have always lived within a society that accepts gender diversity and who have aged within that context, (ii) those who have 'come out' as trans in later life and (iii) those who came out as trans in early life and have since aged. In practice, the delineation between those trajectories is unlikely to be absolute. Given the impact of globalising and colonising influences on state approaches to gender diversity, it may be more common for older people to have had to navigate and integrate different cultural perspectives on gender rather than having lived their lives exclusively interacting with a sociocultural setting that recognises and affirms gender diversity. The distinction between trajectory (ii) and (iii) is inevitably a gradient rather than an absolute cut off. Nonetheless, this model is useful in considering the interactions between life course, gendered experience and social reactions. For example, some older people will have faced challenges related to gender diversity throughout much of their adult life (but alongside that, perhaps also developed resiliencies and social support to help navigate those challenges). Others may be experiencing such issues for the first time as they are ageing. Some older people may also be dealing with the ways in which ageing impacts upon their existing approaches to navigating life as a trans person, for example that new health needs make it harder to keep aspects of their body private. In Chapter 8, Castle and Kimberly elaborate on the ways in which ageing impacts on the life experiences of trans older people across social care and healthcare settings.

Pearce (2018a) also highlights the impact different trajectories may have upon understandings of age and ageing. Life as a trans person involves understanding and navigating trans-specific issues such as medicolegal structures and dealing with discriminations. Trans people may locate their age both in terms of their total lifespan and the time they have been interacting with the world as a trans person. In some senses, therefore, a 30-year-old who transitioned a decade ago may be seen as 'older' than a 60-year-old who is transitioning now. In a related manner, those who transition later in life may emphasise the extent to which this is a rejuvenating experience and may use terminology such as a 'second adolescence' to denote the extent to which transition constitutes a disjunct within the life trajectory (Bailey, 2012; Fabbre, 2014).

Over this, we can also layer the shifting tides of social acceptance. As Kit Heyam explores in more detail in Chapter 10, people undergoing gender transition have been the topic of public debate and media coverage for many decades. However, at present there is a highly charged 'culture war' around gender identity, rights and recognition, and this appears to be having a negative impact upon the mental health of gender diverse people (Hughto et al, 2021; McLean, 2021). Age is sometimes an intersecting component within these debates, for example the claims that the experiences of those who transition in later life are less authentic than those who transition when young (Serano, 2020), or conversely that transitioning in early life represents a form of 'social contagion', in which young people are vulnerable to external influences (Ashley, 2020). While discussing the politics of youth transition is outside the scope of this book, it is worth noting that these debates often implicitly (and sometimes explicitly) position older trans and gender diverse people as suspect.

It is likely that over time the life trajectories of older gender diverse populations will tend to change. As already noted, the demographic trend seems to be towards younger people being more open and visible about gender diverse identities. Over time, this may mean fewer people 'come out' in later life. Perhaps eventually, levels of social acceptance will reach a stage where it does become more common for people to have lived their whole lives outside the gender binary, within a society that is largely accepting. Understanding gender diversity, ageing and the life course is likely to be an ongoing and evolving field of study.

Practical issues in gender diverse ageing

Individuals who first explore and/or express gender diversity in later life often report this to be a joyful experience and indicate an intention to live life to the full (Fabbre, 2014; Willis et al, 2020). However, this may also be tempered with regret that they felt unable to do so earlier (Siverskog, 2015; Willis et al, 2020). Life changes associated with middle or later life, such as retirement, separation and divorce or children reaching adulthood, may facilitate individuals in feeling able to live more openly as trans or non-binary (Jones and Willis, 2016; Willis et al, 2020).

Challenges such as socioeconomic exclusion, discrimination, lack of legal recognition and poor access to healthcare are frequently faced by gender diverse people of all ages (Winter et al, 2016; Kcomt, 2019). However, these challenges may have greater impact in later life, when people may become less able to independently manage challenges and more reliant upon health and social care services (Witten, 2014; Jones and Willis, 2016). Negative experiences may tend be compounded across the life course – for example, those who experienced financial or employment exclusion earlier in their life may be in a more financially precarious situation in later life. Research suggests that older trans adults have poorer physical and mental health, and this appears to be related to issues such as victimisation and stigma within society (Fredriksen-Goldsen et al, 2013). In Chapter 2, Callahan et al outline some of the barriers older trans people experience within healthcare settings. Building on this, Chapter 3 explores the ways in which trans people may navigate the barriers they face in healthcare services. In Chapter 6, Morgan et al consider the perspective of healthcare professionals and their knowledge and confidence in supporting older trans people.

Advanced ageing and loss of independence are often a particular concern for gender diverse people. Of course, all sectors of society worry about issues such as loss of identity in dementia or needing residential care. However, for older trans people these fears are frequently heightened by concerns – often from personal experience – that they will be subject to direct discrimination by service providers or that their personal choices and identity will be disregarded (Witten and Whittle, 2004; Witten, 2014; Jones and Willis, 2016; Baril and Silverman, 2022). For instance, trans people may have concerns about being able to dress and style their hair in line with their gender identity, or about how they will be memorialised after death (Almack, 2018; Willis et al, 2020). In Chapter 12, Almack et al discuss some of the concerns voiced by trans adults in relation to end-of-life care and the complex decision making individuals and their significant others experience at end of life. In Chapter 7, Sofia Smolle considers social workers' perspectives on supporting older trans people, and in Chapter 11 Phil Harper considers how care cultures address gender neutrality. Many gender diverse people have experienced family rejection or breakdown of intimate relationships and hence may be more likely to have troubled relationships with family or be ageing alone (Witten and Eyler, 2016). Gender diverse people may therefore both have reduced expectations of health and care provision and fewer people they can rely on to advocate for their needs. The latter situation may heighten gender diverse people's needs for help from formal service providers when managing care and support needs and disability in old age. In Chapter 4, Hafford-Letchfield et al explore in more depth the literature on family relationships for older trans people, while Chapter 9 considers support for issues of intimate and domestic violence.

Through the accounts and explorations within this book, we have brought together knowledge and experience emerging from the trans and gender diverse ageing population and created a practical resource for professionals, students and educators. We hope that this will facilitate thoughtful discussion, reflection and practical intervention in order to improve the experiences of ageing and later life services for trans, non-binary and gender diverse people.

References

Almack, K. (2018) '"I didn't come out to go back in the closet": ageing and end of life care for older LGBT people', in A. King, K. Almack, Y.-T. Suen and S. Westwood (eds) *Older Lesbian, Gay, Bisexual and Trans People: Minding the Knowledge Gaps*, Abingdon: Routledge, pp 158–71.

American Psychiatric Association (2013) *DSM-5: Diagnostic and Statistical Manual of Mental Disorders*, Arlington: American Psychiatric Association.

Ansara, Y.G. (2012) 'Cisgenderism in medical settings: challenging structural violence through collaborative partnerships', in I. Rivers and R. Ward (eds) *Out of the Ordinary: LGBT Lives*, Newcastle upon Tyne: Cambridge Scholars Publishing, pp 102–22.

Ansara, Y.G. (2015) 'Challenging cisgenderism in the ageing and aged care sector', *Australasian Journal on Ageing*, 34(S2): 14–18.

Ashley, F. (2020) 'A critical commentary on "rapid-onset gender dysphoria"', *The Sociological Review*, 68(4): 779–99.

Bailey, L. (2012) 'Trans ageing', in R. Ward, I. Rivers and M. Sutherland (eds) *Lesbian, Gay, Bisexual and Transgender Ageing: Biographical Approaches for Inclusive Care and Support*, London: Jessica Kingsley Publishers, pp 51–66.

Baril, A. and Silverman, M. (2022) 'Forgotten lives: trans older adults living with dementia at the intersection of cisgenderism, ableism/cogniticism and ageism', *Sexualities*, 25(1–2): 117–31.

Bauer, G.R., Hammond, R., Travers, R., Kaay, M., Hohenadel, K.M. and Boyce, M. (2009) '"I don't think this is theoretical; this is our lives": how erasure impacts health care for transgender people', *The Journal of the Association of Nurses in AIDS Care: JANAC*, 20(5): 348–61.

Fabbre, V.D. (2014) 'Gender transitions in later life: a queer perspective on successful aging', *The Gerontologist*, 55(1): 144–53.

Fredriksen-Goldsen, K.I., Cook-Daniels, L., Kim, H.-J., Erosheva, E.A., Emlet, C.A., Hoy-Ellis, C.P. et al (2013) 'Physical and mental health of transgender older adults: an at-risk and underserved population', *The Gerontologist*, 54(3): 488–500.

Goodman, M., Adams, N., Corneil, T., Kreukels, B., Motmans, J. and Coleman, E. (2019) 'Size and distribution of transgender and gender nonconforming populations: a narrative review', *Endocrinology and Metabolism Clinics*, 48(2): 303–21.

Hughto, J.M., Pletta, D., Gordon, L., Cahill, S., Mimiaga, M.J. and Reisner, S.L. (2021) 'Negative transgender-related media messages are associated with adverse mental health outcomes in a multistate study of transgender adults', *LGBT Health*, 8(1): 32–41.

Human Dignity Trust (2023) 'Map of countries that criminalise LGBT people', London: Human Dignity Trust, Available from: https://www.humandignitytrust.org/lgbt-the-law/map-of-criminalisation/

Jones, S.M. and Willis, P. (2016) 'Are you delivering trans positive care?', *Quality in Ageing and Older Adults*, 17(1): 50–9.

Kcomt, L. (2019) 'Profound health-care discrimination experienced by transgender people: rapid systematic review', *Social Work in Health Care*, 58(2): 201–19.

Lyons, A., Rasmussen, M.L., Anderson, J. and Gray, E. (2021) 'Counting gender and sexual identity in the Australian census', *Australian Population Studies*, 5(1): 40–8.

McLean, C. (2021) 'The growth of the anti-transgender movement in the United Kingdom: the silent radicalization of the British electorate', *International Journal of Sociology*, 51(6): 473–82.

Meier, S.C. and Labuski, C.M. (2013) 'The demographics of the transgender population', in A.K. Baumle (ed) *International Handbook on the Demography of Sexuality*, Dordrecht: Springer, pp 289–327.

Mount, L. (2020) '"I am not a hijra": class, respectability, and the emergence of the "new" transgender woman in India', *Gender & Society*, 34(4): 620–47.

Office for National Statistics (2023) 'Gender identity: age and sex, England and Wales; census 2021', Newport, Available from: https://www.ons.gov.uk/peoplepopulationandcommunity/culturalidentity/genderidentity/articles/genderidentityageandsexenglandandwalescensus2021/2023-01-25

Pearce, R. (2018a) 'Trans temporalities and non-linear ageing', in: A. King, K. Almack, Y.-T. Suen and S. Westwood (eds) *Older Lesbian, Gay, Bisexual and Trans People: Minding the Knowledge Gaps*, Abingdon: Routledge, pp 61–74.

Pearce, R. (2018b) *Understanding Trans Health: Discourse, Power and Possibility*, Bristol: Policy Press.

Ram, A., Kronk, C.A., Eleazer, J.R., Goulet, J.L., Brandt, C.A. and Wang, K.H. (2022) 'Transphobia, encoded: an examination of trans-specific terminology in SNOMED CT and ICD-10-CM', *Journal of the American Medical Informatics Association*, 29(2): 404–10.

Schilt, K. and Bratter, J. (2015) 'From multiracial to transgender? Assessing attitudes toward expanding gender options on the US census', *Transgender Studies Quarterly*, 2(1): 77–100.

Serano, J. (2020) 'Autogynephilia: a scientific review, feminist analysis, and alternative "embodiment fantasies" model', *The Sociological Review*, 68(4): 763–78.

Siverskog, A. (2015) 'Ageing bodies that matter: age, gender and embodiment in older transgender people's life stories', *NORA: Nordic Journal of Feminist and Gender Research*, 23(1): 4–19.

Thelwall, M., Devonport, T.J., Makita, M., Russell, K. and Ferguson, L. (2022) 'Academic LGBTQ+ terminology 1900–2021: increasing variety, increasing inclusivity?', *Journal of Homosexuality*, 70(11): 2514–38.

Towle, E.B. and Morgan, L.M. (2006) 'Romancing the transgender narrative: rethinking the use of the "third gender" concept', in S. Stryker and S. Whittle (eds) *The Transgender Studies Reader*, New York: Routledge, pp 666–84.

Valentine, D. (2007) *Imagining Transgender*, Durham: Duke University Press.

Vincent, B.W. (2018) *Transgender Health*, London: Jessica Kingsley Publishers.

Waling, A., Lyons, A., Alba, B., Minichello, V., Barrett, C., Hughes, M. et al (2019) 'Trans women's perceptions of residential aged care in Australia', *British Journal of Social Work*, 50(5): 1304–23.

Willis, P., Raithby, M., Dobbs, C., Evans, E. and Bishop, J.-A. (2020) '"I'm going to live my life for me": trans ageing, care, and older trans and gender non-conforming adults' expectations of and concerns for later life', *Ageing & Society*, 41(12): 2792–813.

Winter, S., Diamond, M., Green, J., Karasic, D., Reed, T., Whittle, S. et al (2016) 'Transgender people: health at the margins of society', *The Lancet*, 388(10042): 390–400.

Witten, T.M. (2009) 'Graceful exits: intersection of aging, transgender identities, and the family/community', *Journal of GLBT Family Studies*, 5(1–2): 35–61.

Witten, T.M. (2014) 'It's not all darkness: robustness, resilience, and successful transgender aging', *LGBT Health*, 1(1): 24–33.

Witten, T.M. and Eyler, A.E. (2016) 'Care of aging transgender and gender non-conforming patients', in R. Ettner, S. Monstrey and E. Coleman (eds) *Principles of Transgender Medicine and Surgery*, New York: Routledge, pp 344–78.

Witten, T.M. and Whittle, S. (2004) 'Transpanthers: the greying of transgender and the law', *Deakin Law Review*, 9(2): 503–22.

World Health Organization (2023) 'WHO announces the development of a guideline on the health of trans and gender diverse people', Geneva: WHO, Available from: https://www.who.int/news/item/28-06-2023-who-announces-the-development-of-the-guideline-on-the-health-of-trans-and-gender-diverse-people

PART I

What do we know about older trans people's lives and care needs? Messages from research

1

Trans and gender diverse ageing and the life course: what can evidence from quantitative studies tell us about how trans people age?

Dylan Kneale, Evangeline Tabor and Laia Bécares

Introduction

Research exploring LGBTQ+ lives is notably peppered with evidence gaps (King et al, 2018), and this is particularly true for evidence offering insights into the ageing experiences and trajectories of older trans people (Kneale et al, 2021). Much of the existing literature on trans and gender diverse people focuses on younger people's experiences, particularly around medical transition (Willis et al, 2021), and where literature has centred on older trans people's experiences, it has often focused on problematic relationships with healthcare providers and to a lesser extent on relationships with social care or housing providers (King, 2015; Bouman et al, 2016; King and Stoneman, 2017; Willis et al, 2021). Examples that document positive experiences of trans ageing, in addition to experiences of discrimination and exclusion, are much rarer. However, qualitative studies that draw on inductive approaches highlight that many older trans people regard older age as a period to live life to the full (Willis et al, 2021).

Understanding trans people's ageing experiences using quantitative methods can often involve attempting to impose crisp parameters around concepts that are, by their nature, fuzzy, complex and evolving. Callahan (2021) highlights how terminology used to describe trans people has evolved from earlier terms that reflected clothing and appearance to those that reflect more holistic understandings of gender diversity. Our own search for literature in this area drew on Stonewall's (2023) (non-exhaustive) list of 17 terms associated with trans identities, from those with more clinical origins such as transsexual to more encompassing terms such as non-binary (Stonewall, 2023). A second fuzzy concept relates to older people and ageing. Defining people as 'older people' on the basis of their chronological age is conceptually fraught. Population ageing and increases in longevity mean that we now apply the label of 'older person' to 60-year-olds, for example, who may remain in this category for two or three decades, and in doing so we implicitly – and erroneously – assume and ascribe commonalities to this period of life afterwards (Kydd et al, 2018). Evidence from longitudinal studies such as the English Longitudinal Study of Ageing (ELSA), can help to challenge such assumptions, and these studies typically start to monitor expectations and preparations for older age and experiences of ageing among those aged 50 and over (Steptoe et al, 2013). However, such studies are not only constructed with the assumption that there are a set of common, cis-normative, life course markers and experiences, but that these can be measured in a common temporal rubric across groups. Such a rubric may not be applicable or appropriate for understanding trans life course patterns, which may follow their own temporal frames (*trans time*) that do not necessarily involve 'bourgeois reproduction and family, longevity … and inheritance' (Halberstam, 2005, quoted in Pearce, 2018, p 62) and instead involve 'non-linear temporalities of disruption, disjuncture and discontinuity' (Pearce, 2018, p 61). More broadly, due to structural oppression, the health markers of chronological age around frailty and poor health are likely to appear earlier for LGBTQ+ people, and so the process of categorising old age at 60, or even 50, obscures the early onset of poor health for many trans people in later life, and thus underestimates inequalities.

The complexity of applying crisp parameters to complex and fuzzy constructs ties into broader debates and disagreements around the suitability and use of hetero- and cis-normative categories to tell the story of LGBTQ+ people's experiences (see Guyan, 2022, for a comprehensive overview). There are legitimate concerns about the way in which the methods used and decisions made within quantitative analytical frameworks serve to focus attention on the magnitude of impacts while obfuscating their meaning and construction (Guyan, 2022), as well as serving to further erase or marginalise intersectional groups. This is often a reflection of the heterosexism and cisgenderism that leads to poor investment into both the data infrastructure and capacity building for researching trans lives (and LGBTQ+ people's lives more broadly). For example, in illuminating the need for better mental health support for trans and gender diverse people during the COVID-19 pandemic, our own previous research aggregated diverse experiences (including trans men, trans women and non-binary experiences) in a way that could have obfuscated large differences in need between groups; at the same time, we marginalised trans participants' gender and sexuality in a way that we didn't for other LGBTQ+ respondents (see Kneale and Bécares, 2021). These choices were made in the absence of any large-scale focused and funded data collection to understand trans (or indeed LGBTQ+) experiences during the pandemic in the UK. Although the chosen analytical strategy reflected considerations of the conceptual similarities/differences between groups and the numbers across groups within our sample, as well as the decision to adopt an 'inclusive' or 'specific' approach in the analysis (Restar et al, 2020), our decision to aggregate the data in order to surface the need for mental health support for trans people during the COVID-19 pandemic will almost certainly have blurred or even erased the meaning and distinctions of trans participants' identities. With further investment and a strengthened data infrastructure, quantitative data could nevertheless be used in compelling ways to add insight into the processes and sociopolitical context of trans ageing and how these experiences differ across different intersections of identity, gender, ethnicity, class, sexuality and disability. Evidence from quantitative studies could be used to help design more appropriate policy and services and to 'create conditions that enable' older trans people 'to lead full, authentic lives' (Guyan, 2022, p 1).

Nevertheless, our own experiences to date as quantitative researchers examining patterns of LGBTQ+ ageing are that quantitative data that can be used to examine trans lives and trans ageing in the UK have been historically lacking. This dearth can be attributed to several factors. First, gender minorities have been rendered invisible within several large datasets (Kneale et al, 2020). Second, the use of binary gender variables and assumptions of stability in these constructs preclude accurate identification of trans respondents (Bécares, 2020, p 2431). Third, data on sexual and gender minorities are frequently subject to additional restrictions around usage (Tabor et al, 2023). The absence of quantitative data and evidence on trans ageing experiences is particularly concerning given that qualitative evidence can sometimes occupy an uncertain position in public policy making (Kneale et al, 2019), although it is thought to comprise the bulk of research conducted on LGBTQ+ later lives (Kneale et al, 2021).

In this chapter, we aim to cover three elements of quantitative research on trans ageing. First, we briefly explore theories that may be relevant for examining trans ageing that can provide an indication of where quantitative data could and should make a contribution. Second, we examine the potential of existing UK quantitative data to undertake theory-driven research about trans people's ageing trajectories. Finally, we dedicate the majority of the chapter to reviewing what recent UK and international literature can tell us about later life among trans people through conducting a systematic scoping review of recent quantitative evidence. The purpose of this chapter is not to provide a definitive framework of what could and should be collected in future quantitative data collection; such an exercise is beyond the scope of this chapter and should be co-produced with trans people who represent a range of identities, perspectives and intersections. We advocate for co-production as the practice includes a commitment towards creating fairer and more equitable societies through shifting the hierarchies of power away from academics and academic institutions and ensuring research is created in ways that are accessible, inclusive, mutually beneficial and action-orientated

(O'Mara-Eves et al, 2022). Instead, this chapter aims to (i) provide a resource of evidence for when such a co-produced endeavour takes place, and (ii) stimulate interest in quantitative research in trans ageing by highlighting where knowledge has been generated and where gaps remain.

Theoretically driven guidance for quantitative studies

Previous systematic reviews exploring the role of theory in understanding patterns of LGBTQ+ ageing have illustrated that an array of theories have been used in research (quantitative and qualitative) in this area, with minority or social stress (see Brooks, 1981; Meyer, 2003), the health equity promotion model (see Fredriksen-Goldsen et al, 2014b) and theories around resilience (see, for example, Fredriksen-Goldsen, 2007) being those most commonly drawn upon in LGBTQ+ focused social gerontological research (Fabbre et al, 2018).

The Gender Minority Stress Framework (GMSF) is an adaptation of the minority stress framework. The minority stress framework posits that unique social stressors faced by LGBTQ+ people as a minority group indirectly and directly lead to inequalities in health (Meyer, 2003). However, the GMSF acknowledges that the stressors experienced on the basis of being a gender minority are not necessarily the same as those on the basis of being a sexual minority (Testa et al, 2015; Tan et al, 2020a). The framework includes factors reflecting individual and social stressors such as measures of gender-related discrimination, rejection, victimisation, non-affirmation of gender identity, internalised transphobia and non-disclosure of identity, as well as protective factors on the individual level (pride) and community level (community connectedness) (Testa et al, 2015; Tan et al, 2020a). Consideration of the GMSF also introduces a number of related concepts and processes that may be experienced by older trans people including cisnormativity (related to the institutionalised social norm of being cisgender, including situations where people refuse to acknowledge trans identities or experiences), transphobia (processes related to discrimination against trans people) and transmisogyny (reflecting the oppressive intersection between transphobia and misogyny that many transwomen face, which is experienced to a greater degree along intersections of class and ethnicity [Krell, 2017]). While the GMSF acknowledges trans-specific social stressors, critical analysis of the model by Tan and colleagues (2020a) illuminated a need for the GMSF to better account for individuals' intersecting identities and their cultural embeddedness. Incorporating indigenous perspectives and intersectional viewpoints could help to address this need (Tan et al, 2020a). In addition, the GMSF shares some of the same weaknesses as original iterations of the minority stress framework in appearing to underemphasise structural and environmental factors and downplaying resilience-promoting factors.

Theories around resilience have also been adapted to account for resilience-promoting factors experienced by gender minority people. These include the Transgender Resilience Intervention Model, developed to help design and interpret evidence from resilience-promoting interventions, which emphasises the importance of group-level processes (for example, levels of social support, community belonging and activism) as well as individual-level processes (for example, self-worth, self-acceptance and transition) that promote resilience (Matsuno and Israel, 2018). Finally, the Health Equity Promotion Model draws on elements of life course theory and aims to recognise the health-promoting strengths and resources that are specific to sexual and gender minorities, as well as the multifaceted ways in which individual and social factors interact with forms of exclusion and discrimination to impede attaining health equity (Fredriksen-Goldsen et al, 2014b). This model was developed with the explicit purpose of explaining not only why LGBTQ+ people may be more likely to experience health inequities but also why many LGBTQ+ people experience good health across the life course, which counteracts expectations based on the oppression and discrimination they experience (Fredriksen-Goldsen et al, 2014b).

Previous systematic reviews of LGBTQ+ ageing have drawn upon different theoretical frameworks including minority stress (Kneale et al, 2021) but also on life course theory as a framework for understanding the diverse and intersectional ageing trajectories of older LGBTQ+ people (Fredriksen-Goldsen and Muraco, 2010; Fredriksen-Goldsen et al, 2019). Life course theory usually focuses on how the timing, sequence, context, structural location and social construction of roles, milestones and major life transitions take place and differ across groups (Elder, 2003). In adapting a framework based on life course theory, Fredriksen-Goldsen et al (2019) and colleagues developed the Iridescent Life Course as a 'blueprint' for future research. Their Iridescent Life Course framework corroborated established areas of concern in life course theory including the interplay of LGBTQ+ older people's lives with historical and current broader context; the linked and interdependent lives that LGBTQ+ people lead with other LGBTQ+ people and beyond; the importance of the timing and context of LGBTQ+ specific milestones such as identity development, coming out and disclosure experiences; and human agency and the resilience and advocacy that takes place among LGBTQ+ communities (Fredriksen-Goldsen et al, 2019).

At the time of writing, we were unable to identify examples where the Iridescent Life Course framework has been applied to understand patterns of trans ageing specifically, although many of the domains included could feasibly be adapted to better understand older trans' experiences including those tenets reflecting: milestones and identity development; human agency and resilience and advocacy; linked and interdependent lives; and the interplay of older people's lives with historical and current broader context.

Investigations of older trans ageing trajectories are likely to require greater consideration of health and the relationships between older trans people and health and social care providers. Models such as the Transgender Emergence Model and the allied Gender Affirmation framework explicitly make connections between health and social support providers and trans people's outcomes. In the latter, the model explores how 'social oppression decreases access to gender affirmation while psychological distress increases the need for gender affirmation', with gender affirmation entailing support from social support networks as well as gender-affirming healthcare (Sevelius, 2013, p 685). For some trans people who are older, interactions with health and care providers may involve seeking out gender-affirming healthcare and care for age-related chronic conditions simultaneously. However, while existing models and theories consider both the development of trans identity and the societal barriers to living authentically, they seemingly overlook the crucial intersection of trans identity and age-related concerns.

It is clear that there is no unifying framework for theorising ageing patterns and life course trajectories of older trans people; part of this may reflect the heterogeneity of gender minority groups as well as the complexity of theorising life course patterns that may follow non-linear temporalities characterised by disruption and disjuncture (Pearce, 2018). Another likely explanation revolves around the underfunding of research and data infrastructure to understand trans experiences in later life. Others have noted that previous attempts to address this gap appear to have over-problematised ageing experiences and trajectories and indicated a need to understand factors that promote as well as inhibit positive ageing experiences and trajectories among older trans people (Fredriksen-Goldsen et al, 2019). They also point towards a need for understanding experiences at the intersections of age, gender, ethnicity, disability, sexual orientation and class (see Crenshaw, 1991). In the remainder of the chapter, we explore if, and how, existing quantitative evidence has explored these themes. We first outline the potential of existing sources of quantitative data to explore these concerns, with a particular focus on UK datasets.

Observing trans ageing in quantitative datasets

Much of our insight on patterns of ageing in the general population are drawn from large population-level longitudinal datasets such as ELSA and the (US-based) Health and Retirement Survey, although a recent review suggests that these studies and others have inadequate measures to understand patterns of trans ageing (see Hanes and Clouston, 2021). In the case of ELSA, relevant measures appear entirely absent, with a single question on sex asked once in the survey (Hanes and Clouston, 2021), rendering trans participants analytically invisible. This approach is contrary to recommended practice to field two questions that ask separately about sex and gender (Hanes and

Clouston, 2021) and differs from the 2021 census in England and Wales, where two questions were used for the entire population (Office for National Statistics, 2023). This absence could be explained by concerns about the level of non-response among older respondents (and even concerns of attrition) around the fielding of questions of sex and gender in population-based surveys. However, there is little evidence to support these concerns (Fraser et al, 2020), and while there is an increasing pattern of non-response to questions of gender identity with age, levels of non-response nevertheless remain very low (for example, under 1 per cent in a recent sweep of the Behavioral Risk Factor Surveillance System [BRFSS] survey [Cloyes et al, 2016]).

Prior reviews have illustrated limitations in existing UK data sources for studying older trans lives, largely due to the lack of a gender identity question that facilitates identifying trans people. Despite this, there are promising signs that surveys are adopting a more inclusive approach. One example is the UK Household Longitudinal Study (UKHLS, also known as Understanding Society [see Carpenter, 2022]), which in 2020/21 asked participants to report their gender identity in addition to their sex. The level of refusal to questions on gender was similar to that for sex at birth among those aged 50+ (0.13 per cent and 0.10 per cent respectively among respondents who completed the self-completion module). Among participants with valid responses, there were relatively modest numbers of people aged 50+ who could be identified as trans, with only 0.23 per cent (n=29) of respondents identified as trans (authors' own analyses). Clearly, such small numbers preclude undertaking in-depth quantitative analysis to explore questions based on the analytical frameworks described earlier. In addition, the focus of multipurpose surveys such as the UKHLS is neither on ageing and older people nor trans people, limiting their capacity to address research questions deriving from such frameworks.

In contrast, a source of UK evidence with a comparatively large number of older trans respondents is the Government Equalities Office's 'National LGBT Survey' (Government Equalities Office, 2018), a convenience sample of over 108,000 LGBTQ people that included almost 1,000 (n=989) trans people aged 55+ with substantial numbers of trans women (n=636) and non-binary older people (n=197) and smaller numbers of trans men (n=58) and people who identified as another gender minority identity (n=98). Evidence from these data finds that the likelihood of having been resident in a residential, nursing or care home for older people is much higher among trans older people aged 65+ (6.9 per cent) than among cisgender LGB people aged 65+ (where the levels were negligible). Although the survey's design makes it challenging to generalise the findings to the broader population (the survey drew on a convenience sample), this may reflect trans older people having poorer health and/or weaker social support systems that could provide informal care. Other findings from the data specific to older trans people aged 65+ include a twofold higher risk of having received or been offered conversion therapy over the life course relative to older cisgender LGB people (19.8 per cent vs 9.9 per cent). While these data offer some insights into the lives and experiences of older trans people, the survey was not designed to capture the specific experiences of older people, or trans people, and at the time of writing there was no mechanism for undertaking additional secondary data analyses of these data.

The lack of available quantitative data sources that can be used to address research questions relevant for trans ageing, and that include sufficient numbers of participants to undertake meaningful research, may prompt researchers to collect their own quantitative data on older trans people through surveys. While data from such samples have provided some meaningful insights into older trans lives, their comparability with cisgender populations or their representativeness of older trans populations has been uncertain, as has the extent to which they have addressed issues around underrepresentation of intersectional groups (Stall et al, 2016). Much of this uncertainty had derived from the longstanding absence of a representative sampling frame to recruit participants or to inform weighting strategies, as the sociodemographic characteristics of UK older trans people have been unknown. Fortunately, the results of the UK 2021 Census[1] provide some insights into the older trans population, with the results for gender by age already showing some of the differences in identities by age (see Figure 1.1 based on authors' own analyses of data published by Office for National Statistics [2023]). These show that there over 50,000 (approximately 50,795) trans people aged 55+ living in England and Wales, representing 0.27 per cent of the population aged 55+ (0.29 per cent who answered the question on gender). The data also show that among approximately half of older trans people aged 55+ (50.4 per cent), while they report a different gender to their sex, they do not describe their gender through a specific identity or category.

While the census undoubtedly adds valuable insights into the characteristics of the older trans population, issues nevertheless exist with the collection of sex and gender data that mean uncertainties remain. Some of these uncertainties are described in commentaries and responses on the census questions and accompanying guidance on sex and gender questions, as well as media reports from the time (Fugard, 2020; Hines, 2020; i Team, 2021). These illuminate the charged climate in which trans people of all ages were completing the census, which included attempts to stoke fear that a question on gender would replace the question on sex (despite the census clearly asking both questions separately) and a debate that surfaced the voices of some researchers but marginalised communities; in the midst of hostility (and arguably because of the hostility), trans people received mixed messages on how to actually respond to the 2021 census. Therefore, uncertainties remain in the interpretation of the data presented in Figure 1.1. Nevertheless, this preliminary examination of UK census and survey data underscores the lack of a nationally representative

Figure 1.1: Distribution of gender identities among older trans people aged 55+ in England and Wales

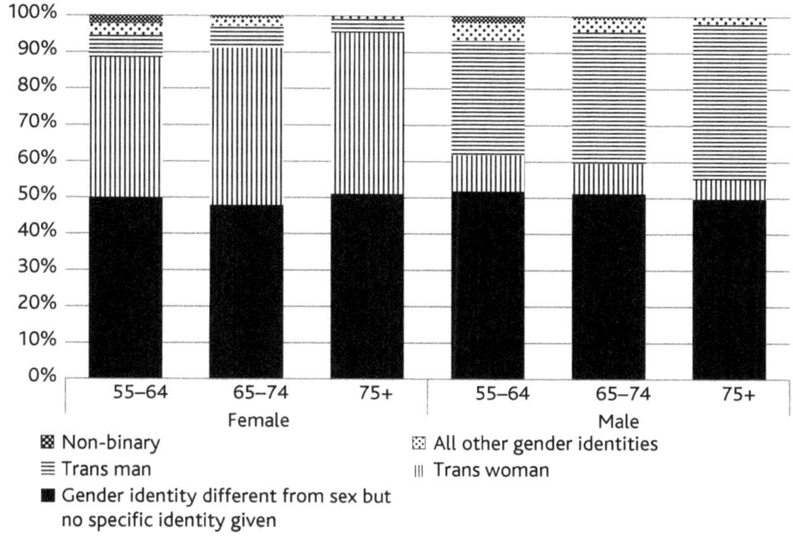

[Stacked bar chart showing percentages across age groups 55–64, 65–74, 75+ for Female and Male, with categories: Non-binary, All other gender identities, Trans man, Trans woman, Gender identity different from sex but no specific identity given]

Note: Columns represent percentage within age group.
Source: Based on Office for National Statistics, 2023, where data on both sex and gender identity provided

dataset in the UK that (i) asks clear, appropriate questions to identify older trans people; (ii) includes a sufficient number of older trans individuals to allow for meaningful quantitative analysis; and (iii) allows for the investigation of pertinent questions grounded in theories of ageing and trans ageing.

There are clear steps that investigators leading nationally representative ageing studies need to take in order to remedy the current analytic invisibility of trans people within data. At the same time, within the UK, other large population-level studies have made attempts to be inclusive of trans identities within their data. Furthermore, and despite the limitations, census data offer a resource for understanding some of the characteristics of older trans people and more accurate assessments of representativeness of future quantitative studies. In the next section, we examine what existing quantitative evidence can tell us about older trans lives and ageing trajectories by presenting the results of a systematic scoping review.

Trans lives and ageing trajectories: evidence from quantitative studies

In this section, we introduce the results of a systematic scoping review that explores the methods (including study design and analytical strategies) and characteristics and results of studies that have used quantitative methods to explore the lives of trans older people or ageing trajectories. The methods for the review are outlined in a protocol published elsewhere (Kneale et al, 2023). Studies were identified as being focused on older trans people and ageing when they: (i) included participants aged 50 and over; (ii) included participants aged 18+ where the mean age of participants was aged 50+; (iii) included participants aged 18+ where differences by age was a focus of the study and data were presented on defined subgroups of older trans people; or (iv) had a self-defined focus on older trans or trans people at midlife or on age-related circumstances or conditions. Studies that focused on LGBTQ+ populations more broadly without a specific focus on trans people were not included.

Overview of publication trends and study designs

A total of 32 studies were identified as meeting the inclusion criteria (see Table 1.1 for an overview). Most studies were conducted among older trans people living exclusively or predominantly within the United States (n=27), with smaller numbers conducted within the UK (n=3), Australia (n=1), Germany (n=1) and New Zealand (n=1). Only one study had conducted a cross-country comparison, with a study conducted by Toze et al (2023) comparing patterns of social support among trans older people in the UK and Australia. Ten studies focused on trans populations aged 50+, with the majority including younger and older participants, albeit retaining a focus on older people and ageing either in terms of the mean age or in terms of the conditions under study. This perhaps emphasises the need for quantitative researchers in this space to adopt less stringent criteria around chronological age when exploring patterns of trans ageing, aligned with different notions of temporality in the life course.

The included studies also point towards increasing interest in using quantitative methods to understand older trans lives over time. The earliest studies were published in the 1980s among trans people recruited from populations who were receiving gender-affirming medical care (Roback et al, 1984; Roback and Lothstein, 1986). After this point, no other studies were identified as using quantitative methods until the 2010s, with Porter et al (2013) publishing a re-analysis of the Trans MetLife Study; thereafter, we identified an uptick in included studies, with five studies included published in 2020 and 2022 respectively.

All the studies adopted a cross-sectional design – no longitudinal study applying quantitative methods to understand trans ageing was identified. A third of the studies made comparisons between trans and cisgender older people (n=10), with the remaining studies drawing on comparisons between different trans identities or between different intersections based on sexuality

Table 1.1: Overview of included study characteristics

Item	Description of main trans population of interest	Criteria around age	Country	Main focus
Bouman et al (2016)	Trans female Trans male	Aged 50+	UK	Sociodemographic and clinical characteristics of patients
Breidenstein et al (2019)	Trans or transgender women/females	Aged 18+ (with mean age 50+)	Germany	Mental health and inequalities
Cai et al (2019)	Trans or transgender women/females Trans or transgender men/males	Aged 18+ (with older subgroup distinguished [60+])	USA	Mental health and inequalities
Cicero et al (2023)	Trans or transgender women/females Trans or transgender men/males Gender non-conforming	Identified as midlife or older (45+)	USA	Cognitive decline
Fredriksen-Goldsen et al (2014a)	Trans or transgender (no gender breakdown)	Aged 50+	USA	Mental health and inequalities; physical health and inequalities
Henry et al (2020)	Gender – masculine Gender – feminine Gender non-conforming Genderqueer Transfeminine Transmasculine	Age 18+ (with a focus on age-related condition)	Primarily USA	Level and types of concerns about ageing; preparedness for ageing
Hillman (2022)	Male to Female Female Trans female Female to male Genderqueer Male Trans male Non-binary	Aged 50+	USA	Experience of intimate partner violence
Howerton and Harris (2022)	Trans or transgender (no gender breakdown)	Age 18+ (with a focus on age related condition)	USA	Physical health and inequalities
Hoy-Ellis et al (2017)	Trans or transgender (no gender breakdown)	Aged 50+	USA	Mental health and inequalities; military service
Jackman et al (2018)	Transfeminine	Aged 18+ (with older subgroup distinguished)	Primarily USA	Mental health and inequalities
Kattari and Hasche (2016)	Male/man Female/woman	Aged 18+ (with older subgroup distinguished: 50–64, 65+)	USA	Experience of stigma

(continued)

Table 1.1: Overview of included study characteristics (continued)

Item	Description of main trans population of interest	Criteria around age	Country	Main focus
Mahowald et al (2021)	Trans or transgender women	Aged 18+ (with mean age 50+)	USA	Physical health and inequalities
Margulies et al (2021)	Male to Female Gender non-conforming Female to male	Aged 18+ (with mean age 50+)	USA	Health service access/support
Marthi et al (2022)	Male to female	Identified as midlife or older (40+)	USA	Physical health and inequalities; health service access/support
Mohamed and Hunter (2019)	Trans or transgender women	Identified as midlife or older (mean age 49)	UK	Level and types of concerns about ageing
Narayan et al (2017)	Male to female Female to male Gender non-conforming	Identified as midlife or older (40+)	USA	Physical health and inequalities; health service access/support
Nokoff et al (2018)	Female to male Male to female Gender non-conforming	Age 18+ (with a focus on age-related condition)	USA	Physical health and inequalities
Porter et al (2013)	Trans or transgender (no gender breakdown)	Aged 50+	Primarily USA	Religiosity; successful ageing or life course markers
Pratt-Chapman and Ward (2020)	Male Female	Identified as midlife or older (40+)	USA	Health service access/support
Roback et al (1984)	Male to female 'Sex change applicant'	Identified as midlife or older (40+)	USA	Sociodemographic and clinical characteristics of patients
Roback and Lothstein (1986)	'Sex change applicant' Transsexual	Identified as midlife or older (40+)	USA	Sociodemographic and clinical characteristics of patients
Seay et al (2017)	Trans or transgender men	Age 18+ (with a focus on age-related condition)	USA	Health service access/support
Stowell et al (2020)	Trans or transgender (no gender breakdown)	Aged 50+	USA	Physical health and inequalities; health service access/support
Tan et al (2020b)	Trans or transgender women Trans or transgender men Non-binary	Aged 18+ (with older subgroup distinguished)	New Zealand	Mental health and inequalities

Table 1.1: Overview of included study characteristics (continued)

Item	Description of main trans population of interest	Criteria around age	Country	Main focus
Tatum et al (2020)	Trans or transgender women Trans or transgender men Genderqueer Assigned female at birth Assigned male at birth	Age 18+ (with a focus on age-related condition)	USA	Successful ageing or life course markers
Toze et al (2023)	Trans or transgender women Trans or transgender men Non-binary (trans non-binary) Gender diverse (no trans background)	Aged 60+	UK Australia	COVID experiences; social support
Walker et al (2017)	Trans or transgender (no gender breakdown) Gender non-conforming	Aged 50+	Primarily USA	Successful ageing or life course markers; health service access/support
Walker et al (2022)	Gender – masculine Gender – feminine Trans or transgender (no gender breakdown) Trans or transgender women Trans or transgender men Genderqueer Other Androgynous Two-spirit	Aged 18+ (with older subgroup distinguished)	Primarily USA	Level and types of concerns about ageing
White Hughto and Reisner (2018)	Female to male Male to female Trans or transgender (no gender breakdown) *Note – breakdown in sample characteristics but not results*	Aged 50+	USA	Mental health and inequalities
Witten (2014)	Transfeminine Androgynous Genderqueer Trans or transgender (no gender breakdown) Trans or transgender women Trans or transgender men Other Two-spirit Third gender Transblended	Aged 18+ (with older subgroup distinguished)	Primarily USA	Successful ageing or life course markers; end-of-life care; preparedness for ageing

(continued)

Table 1.1: Overview of included study characteristics (continued)

Item	Description of main trans population of interest	Criteria around age	Country	Main focus
Witten (2015)	Specific trans subgroup – trans-lesbian	Age 18+ (with a focus on age-related condition)	Primarily USA	End-of-life care; preparedness for ageing;
Witten (2016)	Specific trans subgroup – trans-bisexual	Age 18+ (with a focus on age-related condition)	Primarily USA	Level and types of concerns about ageing; preparedness for ageing; end-of-life care

(for example Witten, 2015), or age (for example Jackman et al, 2018), or other sociodemographic characteristics. Most of the studies appeared to draw upon existing secondary data sources (n=22), including the (predominantly) US-based Trans MetLife Survey on Later-Life Preparedness and Perceptions in Transgender-Identified Individuals (known as TMLS) (n=5: Porter et al, 2013; Witten, 2015, 2016; Walker et al, 2017; Walker et al, 2022); the BRFSS (n=4: Narayan et al, 2017; Stowell et al, 2020; Marthi et al, 2022; Cicero et al, 2023); the Ageing with Pride Study (n=2: Fredriksen-Goldsen et al, 2014a; Hoy-Ellis et al, 2017); the National Transgender Discrimination Survey (n= 2: Kattari and Hasche, 2016; Cai et al, 2019); and the US Transgender Survey (n=2: Tatum et al, 2020; Hillman, 2022). Each of these examples of secondary data analysis underscore the enduring advantages that investments into data on older trans lives can yield. Most other studies featured analyses of surveys specifically designed by the authors to address the research question central to their paper. One exception was the single study that drew on administrative data (clinical records) as the data source (Mahowald et al, 2021). A further four studies also drew on samples recruited from within clinical settings (Roback et al, 1984; Roback and Lothstein, 1986; Bouman et al, 2016; Breidenstein et al, 2019), emphasising the medical orientation of a substantial portion of the literature. Sample sizes varied, from the smallest including just 13 in Roback and Lothstein (1986) to the largest attaining a sample size of almost 3,500 (3,462) older trans people aged 50+ (Hillman, 2022). Sample size often determined the scope of the analytical methods that were employed, and 11 studies relied on descriptive methods (charting the data and, for example, employing bivariate tests of association), while other studies used more complex analytical methods, for example various types of regression and/or multivariate analyses.

Finally, we examined the population of interest. A complex array of identities was measured by researchers (Figure 1.2), with terms around trans or transgender, or simply referring to a gender, being most common. In line with the more clinically oriented studies in the review, a number of studies

Figure 1.2: Distribution of gender identities among quantitative studies of older trans lives and ageing

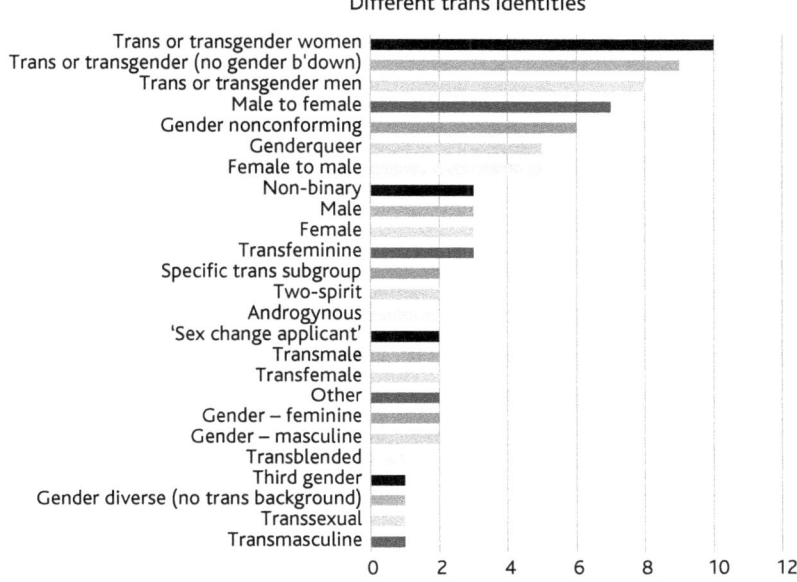

Note: Bars represent number of studies with data on the group.

focused on the 'direction' of the gender-affirming treatment (for example, 'female-to-male').

Insights around physical health and inequalities

Several studies explored physical health trajectories among older trans people, although the evidence base appeared to offer only a fragmented picture. Nevertheless, when compared with cisgender older people, the evidence suggests that older trans people have poorer physical health and higher levels of disability (Fredriksen-Goldsen et al, 2014a). Further exploration of trans identities finds that relative to cisgender older women, trans women may be particularly prone to myocardial infarction and may have riskier patterns of alcohol consumption (although not when compared to cisgender men); no differences were identified in terms of cardiometabolic events and risk factors between trans men and cisgender men (Nokoff et al, 2018); other studies also point towards a high prevalence of risk factors for cardiovascular disease among trans women (Mahowald et al, 2021). Evidence in Howerton and Harris (2022) also suggests that among those assigned female at birth, those identifying as trans were at higher risk of cardiovascular disease, while no such disparity was observed among cis and trans people assigned male at birth. The studies also demonstrate the challenges in terms of evidence around this area, with differing comparison groups used (that is, studies that choose to make comparisons on the basis of gender vs those that compare on the basis of sex at birth), and some studies containing substantial numbers of younger people in some groups (for example Nokoff et al, 2018) potentially distorting the interpretation with regard to age-related conditions. Other studies considered disparities in levels of chronic illness among older trans people, with indications of higher levels of chronic illness among those with a 'feminine gender self-perception' (Witten, 2014).

Insights around mental health, social support and inequalities

Many of the studies that explored mental health were suggestive of high levels of poor mental health among older trans groups. For example, a small study by White Hughto and Reisner (2018) suggested that close to three fifths of older trans people in their sample (55.7 per cent, n=61) met the clinical threshold for depression; other studies also identified high levels of depression and/or anxiety among older trans people (for example, trans women [Mahowald et al, 2021]). Several studies noted that levels of poor mental health were higher among groups of older trans people than cisgender older people (Fredriksen-Goldsen et al, 2014a; Nokoff et al, 2018; Breidenstein et al, 2019; Tan et al, 2020b). However, two studies suggested that older trans people tended to have better mental health than younger trans people (Jackman et al, 2018; Tan et al, 2020b), meaning the inequity with cisgender people may attenuate slightly with age (Tan et al, 2020b), albeit remaining at unacceptably high levels. Among older trans people, some evidence suggested that identity stigma (internalising oppressive societal attitudes and beliefs around stigmatised groups) was associated with higher levels of depressive symptomology and lower quality of life (Hoy-Ellis et al, 2017). The same (US-based) study also found that older trans people with a history of military service had lower levels of depressive symptomology than trans people with no military service history (Hoy-Ellis et al, 2017).

A study by Toze et al (2023) provided insight around social support, indicating that the majority of older trans people reported being part of social support networks and being both recipients and providers of social supports. Three fifths of older trans participants in their study reported providing support during the COVID-19 pandemic (58.3 per cent), although when asked about an emergency contact, around a fifth reported no emergency contact in the UK (22.9 per cent) and Australia (18.4 per cent), indicative of a nontrivial number who appear to be excluded from social relationships.

Finally, one study considered cognitive health among older trans adults, finding that among older trans people from minoritised ethnic groups, the level of self-perceived cognitive decline stood at over a fifth (21.6 per cent) higher than among White older trans people (15 per cent) or among older cisgender people from minoritised ethnic groups (12.0 per cent) or who were White (9 per cent) (Cicero et al, 2023). This study highlights the important insights that result from taking an intersectional approach, which was facilitated in this case by using a large dataset (the BRFSS).

Insights around health service access and barriers

A number of studies examined the relationships between older trans people and healthcare providers, including the extent to which they faced barriers to equitable and affirming healthcare.

In terms of gender-affirming treatment, Bouman and colleagues (2016) explored the profile of attendees at a gender identity clinic service and found that older trans people were more likely to have obtained hormone treatment without medical advice than younger trans people and speculate that ageism and weaker social and socioeconomic support structures could explain this difference. The same study found indications that access to hormones among older transwomen was associated with lower levels of anxiety, with other studies also finding that older trans people reported better quality of life after receiving gender-affirming medical care (Cai et al, 2019). This underscores the importance of access to gender-affirming healthcare for older trans people who need it.

Lower socioeconomic resources may be more likely to create barriers to accessing health services among older trans people than among cisgender older (LGB) people (Fredriksen-Goldsen et al, 2014a). Nokoff et al (2018) also find that transmen in the US were more likely to be uninsured than cisgender men or women (no such difference existed for transwomen). Socioeconomic factors were not the only barrier to accessing healthcare. Some studies also note the issues raised by a lack of health professionals with expertise in trans healthcare. For example, among the participants in Margulies et al (2021), this meant that many older trans people had not met with physicians to discuss gender-affirming surgery, although the majority were interested in doing so. In Fredriksen-Goldsen et al (2014a), two fifths of older trans people reported fears in accessing health services outside the 'LGBTQ+ community', which was a significant mediator in explaining instances of poorer physical health, disability, depressive symptomology and perceived stress. Similarly, Walker et al (2017) find that confidence that healthcare professionals will treat older trans people with dignity and respect as a trans person was associated with an increased odds of participants feeling they were ageing successfully. While the concept of successful ageing is problematic and can overlook individual patterns of ageing and the diversity and agency in how different groups age, this evidence nevertheless illuminates the importance of access to appropriate and specialist healthcare in supporting the wellbeing of older trans people.

Finally, a number of studies explored potential barriers that older trans people faced in accessing screening services for noncommunicable diseases. The results provide a complex picture, with some studies providing evidence that trans people may be less likely to access certain types of screenings (for example, lung cancer [Stowell et al, 2020]) and to receive recommendations to undertake screening for certain cancers (Pratt-Chapman and Ward, 2020). In contrast, other studies find little difference in screening rates between trans people and cisgender people, for example in the case of mammography (Narayan et al, 2017) and for prostate cancer screening recommendations (Marthi et al, 2022). Previous negative interactions with healthcare providers were also found to shape preferences around how routine screening for age-related conditions should be conducted (Seay et al, 2017).

Insights around stigma and violence

Frameworks around gender minority stress provide a basis for exploring stigmatising behaviours, and a small number of studies provide evidence that older trans people are more likely to have experienced discrimination and victimisation across the life course (Fredriksen-Goldsen et al, 2014b; White Hughto and Reisner, 2018). Older trans people report on average almost twice as many incidents of discrimination and victimisation (an average of 11 across the life course) as older cisgender sexual minority people (six incidents) (Fredriksen-Goldsen et al, 2014a). Such incidents occur within partnerships, with 56.7 per cent of older trans respondents reporting lifetime experience of intimate partner violence in a large study by Hillman (2022). The evidence around how experiences of discrimination vary with age tends to suggest that older people report lower levels, although the evidence is not conclusive or consistent across all contexts (Kattari and Hasche, 2016) and may also be influenced by older people's reluctance to report violence in relationships.

Insights around ageing and preparedness

Witten (2014) finds that many trans people express concern about growing older, with a quarter of trans respondents expressing high levels of concern about their ability to function independently because there would be nobody to care for them, and almost two fifths believing that being trans would mean they would be unlikely to be treated with dignity and respect at the end of their lives. Similar levels of concern were found among studies examining particular intersections of trans people including lesbian trans people (Witten, 2015) and bisexual trans people (Witten, 2016). Despite expressing substantial concern about their future, many trans individuals demonstrated a low level of preparedness for it. Almost three fifths (59.5 per cent) reportedly had no pension or other retirement plans according to a study by Witten (2014). A similar trend was observed in another study by Henry et al (2020), where 70.8 per cent of adult trans respondents stated they were not saving for a pension; the authors speculated that trans adults had more immediate concerns which superseded concerns about ageing (Henry et al, 2020).

Although the evidence suggests high levels of concerns about ageing and low levels of preparedness, the evidence was by no means universally bleak. Echoing some of the findings earlier from qualitative studies where older trans people viewed ageing in positive terms, a study by Porter et al (2013) showed that almost three quarters of older trans participants believed they were ageing 'successfully' (73.4 per cent) among a sample of almost 300 trans people in the United States, despite experiencing considerable levels of disability and chronic illness (29.4 per cent and 34.6 per cent respectively).

Conclusion

Our explorations in this chapter underscore the value that quantitative data can bring to understanding trans ageing trajectories. In particular, the many examples of secondary data analysis – the use and reuse of existing investments in quantitative survey data – demonstrate the value that large sources of data on older trans can bring to the evidence base. It is therefore particularly disappointing that previous large-scale efforts at collecting data from UK older trans people through the 'National LGBT Survey' have not been made available for reuse and reanalysis. The results also illuminate some contradictory patterns in the evidence base, for example around screening, that indicate the need for more concerted and focused systematic review research to explore discrepant evidence further.

This chapter reveals a number of gaps and opportunities in applying quantitative methods to understand the lives of older trans people and ageing trajectories. There is a clear need for longitudinal research to understand trans life course trajectories – the absence of any longitudinal study in the scoping review we have presented in this chapter was striking. The absence of longitudinal data means that we are unable to explore crucial questions that emerge from the evidence, for example why older trans people may have better mental health than younger trans people (Jackman et al, 2018) and the extent to which this is an age, cohort or period effect. There also appear to be substantial knowledge gaps around core topics of interest in social gerontology, including in terms of housing, loneliness, social networks, wealth and retirement. Additionally, drawing on the theoretical frameworks outlined earlier in the chapter, there appear to be gaps in terms of life course markers and transitions, health-promoting factors, as well as in terms of activism and volunteering. In terms of the relationship between older trans people and broader contextual factors, it was striking that only one study focused on older trans experiences during the COVID pandemic using quantitative methods was identified, and no study was identified that focused on other contextual forces that may shape older trans lives including the continued neoliberal pursuit of austerity in (UK) public policy and the cost-of-living crisis. In terms of geographic representativeness, as UK-based researchers we were also struck by the US bias in the literature, with only a small number of studies focused on older trans people conducted in the UK or in any non-US setting, with studies conducted in low and middle income countries absent.

The findings presented here come with certain caveats regarding the execution of the scoping review, particularly the possibility of overlooking some quantitative studies due to narrow search parameters. In addition, the inclusion criteria, which stipulated that the underlying theory and main research question(s) of included studies had to be focused on older trans people, may mean that studies that offer insights on trans lives from other studies focused on older LGBTQ people more broadly are not represented (for example Dickson et al (2021)). Despite these potential limitations, the identified gaps likely hold significance. They underscore the disparity between theoretical understandings of ageing in trans individuals and the actual empirical (quantitative) evidence available. We also note that in addition to addressing the gaps outlined earlier, there is a need to adopt an intersectional lens in exploring these and in particular to understand how older trans lives are shaped by class, ethnicity and disability. Finally, we stress the importance of not exclusively examining these gaps through a 'deficit' lens. Older trans individuals could, for example, experience lower levels of loneliness, more stable housing histories, stronger social networks and residence in supportive communities and localities, although these aspects and processes cannot be empirically quantified without investments in improved co-produced quantitative research. Maintaining this perspective also aligns with calls for researchers to counterbalance the 'joy deficit' often characteristic of the study of trans lives with a more nuanced treatment that also explores the joyful elements of trans identities (Shuster and Westbrook, 2022).

Note

[1] With results currently only available for England and Wales.

References

Bécares, L. (2020) 'Health and socioeconomic inequalities by sexual orientation among older women in the UK: findings from the UK Household Longitudinal Study', *Ageing and Society*, 41(10): 2416–34.

Bouman, W.P., Claes, L., Marshall, E., Pinner, G.T., Longworth, J., Maddox, V. et al (2016) 'Sociodemographic variables, clinical features, and the role of preassessment cross-sex hormones in older trans people', *Journal of Sexual Medicine*, 13(4): 711–19.

Breidenstein, A., Hess, J., Hadaschik, B., Teufel, M. and Tagay, S. (2019) 'Psychosocial resources and quality of life in transgender women following gender-affirming Surgery', *Journal of Sexual Medicine*, 16(10): 1672–80.

Brooks, V.R. (1981) *Minority Stress and Lesbian Women*, Lexington, MA, USA: Lexington Books.

Cai, X., White Hughto, J.M., Reisner, S.L., Pachankis, J.E. and Levy, B.R. (2019) 'Benefit of gender-affirming medical treatment for transgender elders: later-life alignment of mind and body', *LGBT Health*, 6(1): 34–9.

Callahan, E. (2021) '"That's the sick trans person": negotiations, healthcare, and the tension of demedicalization', PhD thesis, Brunel University London.

Carpenter, H. (2022) 'UK Household Longitudinal Study Wave 12 technical report', Colchester, Essex: Institute for Social and Economic Research, University of Essex.

Cicero, E.C., Lett, E., Flatt, J.D., Benson, G.P. and Epps, F. (2023) 'Transgender adults from minoritized ethnoracial groups in the U.S. report greater subjective cognitive decline', *Journals of Gerontology: Series B; Psychological Sciences and Social Sciences*, 78(6): 1051–9.

Cloyes, K., Yang, R. and Latimer, S. (2016) 'Refusal to respond to BRFSS sexual orientation and transgender survey items among adults age 60+', *The Gerontologist*, 56(3):438 438.

Crenshaw, K.W. (1991) 'Mapping the margins: intersectionality, identity politics, and violence against women of color', *Stanford Law Review*, 43(6): 1241–99.

Dickson, L., Bunting, S., Nanna, A., Taylor, M., Hein, L. and Spencer, M. (2021) 'Appointment of a healthcare power of attorney among older lesbian, gay, bisexual, transgender, and queer (LGBTQ) adults in the southern United States', *American Journal of Hospice and Palliative Medicine*, 38(11): 1291–8.

Elder, G.H. and Johnson, M.K. (2003) 'The life course and aging: challenges, lessons, and new directions', in R. Settersten (ed) *Invitation to the Life Course: Towards New Understandings of Later Life* (1st edn), Amityville: Routledge, pp 49–81.

Fabbre, V., Jen, S. and Fredriksen-Goldsen, K. (2018) 'The state of theory in LGBTQ aging: Implications for Gerontological Scholarship', *Research in Aging*, 41(5): 495–518.

Fraser, G., Bulbulia, J., Greaves, L.M., Wilson, M.S. and Sibley, C.G. (2020) 'Coding responses to an open-ended gender measure in a New Zealand national sample', *The Journal of Sex Research*, 57(8): 979–86.

Fredriksen-Goldsen, K.I. (2007) 'HIV/AIDS caregiving: predictors of well-being and distress', *Journal of Gay & Lesbian Social Services*, 18(3–4): 53–73.

Fredriksen-Goldsen, K.I. and Muraco, A. (2010) 'Aging and sexual orientation: a 25-year review of the literature', *Research on Aging*, 32(3): 372–413.

Fredriksen-Goldsen, K.I., Jen, S. and Muraco, A. (2019) 'Iridescent life course: LGBTQ aging research and blueprint for the future; a systematic review', *Gerontology*, 65(3): 253–74.

Fredriksen-Goldsen, K.I., Cook-Daniels, L., Kim, H.J., Erosheva, E.A., Emlet, C.A., Hoy-Ellis, C.P. et al (2014a) 'Physical and mental health of transgender older adults: an at-risk and underserved population', *The Gerontologist*, 54(3): 488–500.

Fredriksen-Goldsen, K.I., Simoni, J.M., Kim, H.-J., Lehavot, K., Walters, K.L., Yang, J. et al (2014b) 'The health equity promotion model: reconceptualization of lesbian, gay, bisexual, and transgender (LGBT) health disparities', *American Journal of Orthopsychiatry*, 84(6): 653–63.

Fugard, A. (2020) 'Should trans people be postmodernist in the streets but positivist in the spreadsheets? A reply to Sullivan', *International Journal of Social Research Methodology*, 23(5): 525–31.

Government Equalities Office (2018) 'National LGBT survey', Government Equalities Office.

Guyan, K. (2022) *Queer Data: Using Gender, Sex and Sexuality Data for Action*, London: Bloomsbury Academic.

Hanes, D.W. and Clouston, S.A. (2021) 'Ask again: including gender identity in longitudinal studies of aging', *The Gerontologist*, 61(5): 640–9.

Henry, R.S., Perrin, P.B., Coston, B.M. and Witten, T.M. (2020) 'Transgender and gender non-conforming adult preparedness for aging: concerns for aging, and familiarity with and engagement in planning behaviors', *International Journal of Transgender Health*, 21(1): 58–69.

Hillman, J. (2022) 'Lifetime prevalence of intimate partner violence and health-related outcomes among transgender adults aged 50 and older', *The Gerontologist*, 62(2): 212–22.

Hines, S. (2020) 'Counting the cost of difference: a reply to Sullivan', *International Journal of Social Research Methodology*, 23(5): 533–8.

Howerton, I. and Harris, J.K. (2022) 'Transgender identity and cardiovascular disease', *Transgender Health*, 7(5): 407–15.

Hoy-Ellis, C.P., Shiu, C., Sullivan, K.M., Kim, H.J., Sturges, A.M. and Fredriksen-Goldsen, K.I. (2017) 'Prior military service, identity stigma, and mental health among transgender older adults', *The Gerontologist*, 57(1): S63–S71.

i Team (2021) 'Judge says trans-inclusive census guidance must be torn up in "legal sex" dispute', *inews*. Available from: https://inews.co.uk/news/uk/judge-trans-inclusive-census-guidance-torn-up-legal-sex-dispute-906669

Jackman, K.B., Dolezal, C. and Bockting, W.O. (2018) 'Generational differences in internalized transnegativity and psychological distress among feminine spectrum transgender people', *LGBT Health*, 5(1): 54–60.

Kattari, S.K. and Hasche, L. (2016) 'Differences across age groups in transgender and gender non-conforming people's experiences of health care discrimination, harassment, and victimization', *Journal of Aging and Health*, 28(2): 285–306.

King, A. (2015) 'Prepare for impact? Reflecting on knowledge exchange work to improve services for older LGBT people in times of austerity', *Social Policy and Society*, 14(1): 15–27.

King, A. and Stoneman, P. (2017) 'Understanding SAFE housing: putting older LGBT★ people's concerns, preferences and experiences of housing in England in a sociological context', *Housing, Care and Support*, 20(3): 89–99.

King, A., Almack, K., Suen, Y.-T. and Westwood, S. (eds) (2018) *Older Lesbian, Gay, Bisexual and Trans People: Minding the Knowledge Gaps*, London: Routledge.

Kneale, D. and Bécares, L. (2021) 'Discrimination as a predictor of poor mental health among LGBTQ+ people during the COVID-19 pandemic: cross-sectional analysis of the online Queerantine study', *BMJ Open*, 11(6): e049405.

Kneale, D., Rojas-García, A. and Thomas, J. (2019) 'Obstacles and opportunities to using research evidence in local public health decision-making in England', *Health Research Policy and Systems*, 17(61).

Kneale, D., Tabor, E. and Bécares, L. (2023) 'Trans and gender diverse ageing and the life course: protocol for a rapid scoping review', London: EPPI Centre, UCL.

Kneale, D., Thomas, J. and French, R. (2020) 'Inequalities in health and care among lesbian, gay and bisexual people aged 50 and over in the United Kingdom: a meta-analysis of individual participant data', *The Journals of Gerontology: Series B; Psychological Sciences and Social Sciences*, 75(8): 1758–71.

Kneale, D., Henley, J., Thomas, J. and French, R. (2021) 'Inequalities in older LGBT people's health and care needs in the United Kingdom: a systematic scoping review', *Ageing & Society*, 41(3): 493–515.

Krell, E.C. (2017) 'Is transmisogyny killing trans women of color? Black trans feminisms and the exigencies of White femininity', *Transgender Studies Quarterly*, 4(2): 226–42.

Kydd, A., Fleming, A., Gardner, S. and Hafford-Letchfield, T. (2018) 'Ageism in the third age', in L. Ayalon and C. Tesch-Römer (eds) *Contemporary Perspectives on Ageism*, Dordrecht: Springer, pp 115–30.

Mahowald, M.K., Maheshwari, A.K., Lara-Breitinger, K.M., Adel, F.W., Pellikka, P.A., Davidge-Pitts, C.J. et al (2021) 'Characteristics of transgender women referred to women's heart clinic', *American Journal of Preventive Cardiology*, 7.

Margulies, I.G., Chuang, C., Travieso, R., Zhu, V., Persing, J.A., Steinbacher, D.M. et al (2021) 'Preferences of transgender and gender-nonconforming persons in gender-confirming surgical care: a cross-sectional study', *Annals of Plastic Surgery*, 86(1): 82–8.

Marthi, S., O'Rourke, T.K., Tucci, C., Pareek, G. and Hyams, E. (2022) 'The state of PSA counseling in male-to-female transgender patients in the US', *Prostate*, 82(14): 1315–21.

Matsuno, E. and Israel, T. (2018) 'Psychological interventions promoting resilience among transgender individuals: transgender resilience intervention model (TRIM)', *The Counseling Psychologist*, 46(5): 632–55.

Meyer, I.H. (2003) 'Prejudice, social stress, and mental health in lesbian, gay, and bisexual populations: conceptual issues and research evidence', *Psychological Bulletin*, 129(5): 674–97.

Mohamed, S. and Hunter, M.S. (2019) 'Transgender women's experiences and beliefs about hormone therapy through and beyond mid-age: an exploratory UK study', *International Journal of Transgenderism*, 20(1): 98–107.

Narayan, A., Lebron-Zapata, L. and Morris, E. (2017) 'Breast cancer screening in transgender patients: findings from the 2014 BRFSS survey', *Breast Cancer Research and Treatment*, 166(3): 875–9.

Nokoff, N.J., Scarbro, S., Juarez-Colunga, E., Moreau, K.L. and Kempe, A. (2018) 'Health and cardiometabolic disease in transgender adults in the United States: Behavioral Risk Factor Surveillance System 2015', *Journal of the Endocrine Society*, 2(4): 349–60.

O'Mara-Eves, A., Laidlaw, L., Candy, B., Vigurs, C., Collis, A. and Kneale, D. (2022) 'The Value of Co-production Research Project: a rapid critical review of the evidence', London: Co-production Collective, UCL.

Office for National Statistics (ONS) (2023) 'Gender identity (8 categories) by age and sex, England and Wales: census 2021', *ONS website* Available from: https://www.ons.gov.uk/peoplepopulationandcommunity/culturali dentity/genderidentity/articles/genderidentityageandsexenglandandwale scensus2021/2023-01-25

Pearce, R. (2018) 'Trans temporalities and non-linear ageing', in A. King, K. Almack, Y.-T. Suen and S. Westwood (eds) *Older Lesbian, Gay, Bisexual and Trans People: Minding the Knowledge Gaps*, London: Routledge, pp 61–74.

Porter, K.E., Ronneberg, C.R. and Witten, T.M. (2013) 'Religious affiliation and successful aging among transgender older adults: findings from the Trans MetLife Survey', *Journal of Religion, Spirituality and Aging*, 25(2): 112–38.

Pratt-Chapman, M.L. and Ward, A.R. (2020) 'Provider recommendations are associated with cancer screening of transgender and gender-nonconforming people: a cross-sectional urban survey', *Transgender Health*, 5(2): 80–5.

Restar, A., Jin, H. and Operario, D. (2020) 'Gender-inclusive and gender-specific approaches in trans health research', *Transgender Health*, 6(5): 235–9.

Roback, H.B. and Lothstein, L.M. (1986) 'The female mid-life sex change applicant: a comparison with younger female transsexuals and older male sex change applicants', *Archives of Sexual Behavior*, 15: 401–15.

Roback, H.B., Felleman, E.S. and Abramowitz, S.I. (1984) 'The mid-life male sex-change applicant: a multiclinic survey', *Archives of Sexual Behavior*, 13(2): 141–53.

Seay, J., Ranck, A., Weiss, R., Salgado, C., Fein, L. and Kobetz, E. (2017) 'Understanding transgender men's experiences with and preferences for cervical cancer screening: a rapid assessment survey', *LGBT Health*, 4(4): 304–9.

Sevelius, J.M. (2013) 'Gender affirmation: a framework for conceptualizing risk behavior among transgender women of color', *Sex Roles*, 68(11–12): 675–89.

Shuster, S.M. and Westbrook, L. (2022) 'Reducing the joy deficit in sociology: a study of transgender joy', *Social Problems*.

Stall, R., Matthews, D.D., Friedman, M.R., Kinsky, S., Egan, J.E., Coulter, R.W. et al (2016) 'The continuing development of health disparities research on lesbian, gay, bisexual, and transgender individuals', American Public Health Association.

Steptoe, A., Breeze, E., Banks, J. and Nazroo, J. (2013) 'Cohort profile: the English longitudinal study of ageing', *International Journal of Epidemiology*, 42(6): 1640–8.

Stonewall (2023) 'List of LGBTQ+ terms', *Stonewall website*, Available from: https://www.stonewall.org.uk/list-lgbtq-terms

Stowell, J.T., Parikh, Y., Tilson, K. and Narayan, A.K. (2020) 'Lung cancer screening eligibility and utilization among transgender patients: an analysis of the 2017–2018 United States Behavioral Risk Factor Surveillance System survey', *Nicotine and Tobacco Research*, 22(12): 2164–9.

Tabor, E., Kneale, D. and Patalay, P. (2023) 'Sexual identity data collection and access in UK population-based studies', *The Lancet Public Health*, 8(6): e400–e401.

Tan, K.K.H., Treharne, G.J., Ellis, S.J., Schmidt, J.M. and Veale, J.F. (2020a) 'Gender minority stress: a critical review', *Journal of Homosexuality*, 67(10): 1471–89.

Tan, K.K.H., Ellis, S.J., Schmidt, J.M., Byrne, J.L. and Veale, J.F. (2020b) 'Mental health inequities among transgender people in Aotearoa New Zealand: findings from the Counting Ourselves survey', *International Journal of Environmental Research and Public Health*, 17(8): 2862.

Tatum, A.K., Catalpa, J., Bradford, N.J., Kovic, A. and Berg, D.R. (2020) 'Examining identity development and transition differences among binary transgender and genderqueer nonbinary (GQNB) individuals', *Psychology of Sexual Orientation and Gender Diversity*, 7(4): 379–85.

Testa, R.J., Habarth, J., Peta, J., Balsam, K. and Bockting, W. (2015) 'Development of the gender minority stress and resilience measure', *Psychology of Sexual Orientation and Gender Diversity*, 2(1): 65–77.

Toze, M., Gates, T.G., Hughes, M., Dune, T., Westwood, S., Hafford-Letchfield, T. et al (2023) 'Social support in older transgender and gender diverse communities in the United Kingdom and Australia: a comparative study during COVID-19', *Journal of Gerontological Social Work*, 66(3): 381–99.

Walker, R.V., Powers, S.M. and Witten, T.M. (2017) 'Impact of anticipated bias from healthcare professionals on perceived successful aging among transgender and gender nonconforming older adults', *LGBT Health*, 4(6): 427–33.

Walker, R.V., Powers, S.M. and Witten, T.M. (2022) 'Transgender and gender diverse people's fear of seeking and receiving care in later life: a multiple method analysis', *Journal of Homosexuality*, 70(14): 3374–98 .

White Hughto, J.M. and Reisner, S.L. (2018) 'Social context of depressive distress in aging transgender adults', *Journal of Applied Gerontology*, 37(12): 1517–39.

Willis, P., Raithby, M., Dobbs, C., Evans, E. and Bishop, J.-A. (2021) '"I'm going to live my life for me": trans ageing, care, and older trans and gender non-conforming adults' expectations of and concerns for later life', *Ageing & Society*, 41(12): 2792–813.

Witten, T.M. (2014) 'End of life, chronic illness, and trans-identities', *Journal of Social Work in End-of-Life & Palliative Care*, 10(1): 34–58.

Witten, T.M. (2015) 'Elder transgender lesbians: exploring the intersection of age, lesbian sexual identity, and transgender identity', *Journal of Lesbian Studies*, 19(1): 73–89.

Witten, T.M. (2016) 'Aging and transgender bisexuals: exploring the intersection of age, bisexual sexual identity, and transgender identity', *Journal of Bisexuality*, 16(1): 58–80.

2

"I need to get on with it": experiences of older trans people navigating healthcare

Evelyn Callahan, Ben Vincent and Richard Holti

Introduction

In 2018, the National Institute for Health Research funded three national projects focusing on questions of trans healthcare in the UK. One of these was the Integrating Care for Trans Adults (ICTA) project, based at the Open University and conducted in collaboration with Yorkshire Mesmac and LGBT Foundation. This project included a national survey that gathered 2,056 responses, one of the largest surveys on trans adults to have taken place in the UK. This survey was used as a screening tool to invite participants to be interviewed, with over 800 individuals volunteering. Participants were purposively selected to explore how specific intersections could shape experiences of trans healthcare, which included Black trans people and trans people of colour, trans people living in rural areas, trans people with low incomes/educational attainment, disabled/chronically ill trans people and older trans people. While we use 'older' as a very broad term, we are referring here to participants aged between 51 and 82 years old. The data reported here include semi-structured interviews with 33 trans people living in the UK; nine were in their 50s, 15 in their 60s, eight in their 70s and one in their 80s at the time of the interview. The overall 'younger' age of this sample means that there is less information about the experiences of healthcare in older age, such as increasing physical frailty, dementia, experiences of social care and so on. These findings are further limited by the study being based on a majority White sample. Participants are described using their age at the time of the interview as well as their gender as they described it. It is important to highlight the experiences of this group as they face unique health challenges, both with transition- and non-transition-related care.

These interviews were conducted between February 2020 and January 2021. Most of the interviews were carried out by trans researchers, who frequently identified where follow-up questioning could lead to richer data on user experiences. Interviews typically lasted between one and three hours and were primarily carried out online. Thematic analysis was used, with at least two researchers (at least one of them trans) coding each interview. Accountability to trans communities was central to the ethos of this project. A patient and public involvement (PPI) group was recruited, composed entirely of trans people with a diversity of experiences and intersections, who reviewed and approved the survey, the interview protocols, the analysis and final reporting of the project.

In this chapter, we will lay out the findings of this subset of the ICTA study. We begin by considering older trans people's experiences of waiting for healthcare, in some cases for years. This is followed by discussions of hormone replacement therapy (HRT), screenings, hair removal and surgery in this population. While these types of care are relevant to people of all ages, these sections highlight the unique needs of, and challenges faced by, older trans people. Finally, we relate participants' experiences of transitioning later in life, concluding with lessons for how best to provide care to this population.

Waiting

Long wait times for transition-related healthcare in the UK immerse trans people in uncertainty and exacerbate poor mental health (Pearce, 2018). While these long waiting times have impacted most participants, older trans people provide a unique perspective. As one participant succinctly put it: "I'm well past the halfway point in my estimated life. I need to get on with it" (woman, aged 71). This can be understood through Vanessa D. Fabbre's framework of 'time served' (before transition) versus 'time left'. This 'awareness of time and the meaning given to its finitude can be a catalyst for looking back, looking forward, and pushing gender identity development into the foreground of one's later life' (2014, p 170). These people are experiencing waiting at a stage of their life where time feels particularly precious. For many, this comes after years of 'time served' waiting to make the decision to transition which makes accessing transition-related care feel particularly urgent for them:

> 'Yes. I thought "great". But then I came to realise about the waiting lists, so it took a lot to get me to the point where I was going to [transition], I had constructed very strong defences against it. And it took a kind of semi-catastrophe to eventually compel me to do it. But anyway, once I had suddenly come to my senses and realised what was going on and what I needed to do, I was really in a hurry. Of course I was.' (Gender non-conforming woman, aged 67)

Another participant expressed a similar sense of urgency:

> 'My mum died when she was 66 and three quarters, and my granddad died at 47. I don't know how long I've got. None of us do. But you

know, I'm at an age now where I'm looking back more than I'm looking forward. So I would like to think that when somebody of advancing years comes forward and says "look, you know, I've been miserable for the last 59 years, I'd like to live out my life as the person that I really am", they would sit up and say "yeah OK, we'll do what we can right away". Rather than saying "oh well, you've got to wait behind all the 18-year-olds". They've got another 60 years to live, you know. Hang on a minute, that ain't fair. I've worked all my life, paid in all my life, I expect something back.' (Transgender woman, aged 61)

This participant is expressing an individualised frustration which may be problematised because younger trans people also struggle with waiting times and face specific barriers and challenges. This can be understood, however, in the context of the systemic failure of trans healthcare services and the age-specific sense of urgency for transition that may manifest a sense of injustice at young people 'skipping the queue', regardless of how long individuals may have been on a waiting list.

Many older participants described accelerating their transition timelines (for example, through accessing private healthcare) or wishing they could. This was in relation to many factors but mainly a sense of 'not having much time left' as well as having a confident understanding of oneself in older age and feeling capable of making these decisions.[1] However, this experience of delayed transition followed by rapid (attempted) progress can be fraught:

'By the fourth [assessment] I was back to the first [doctor]. In his report he reckoned that I was too slow deciding to transition, because of my age. Then in another report he reckoned I was too fast deciding to transition because it only took a year from deciding, to going full time.' (Woman, aged 71)

This is illustrative of how the expectations of Gender Identity Clinic (GIC) practitioners – both when a person transitions (younger) and at what rate (slowly) – can be used to police patients. The GIC demonstrates a lack of cultural competence with understanding why either of these factors may vary, particularly for older people.

This is an example of what happens when an individual does not fit the transnormative (Riggs et al, 2019) model of an acceptable trans patient. Clinical confidence in trans realities is cisnormatively determined. In her analysis of trans temporality, Pearce highlights how in relation to the historic, pathologising logic of trans healthcare, '"wrongness" resides not simply in the body of the individual, but also within limited, conditional discourses of trans possibility, stories of institutional cisgenderism and transphobia, and knowledge of the long waits for treatment' (2018, p 127). It's important for clinicians to consider trans temporality (that is, the significance of how a person's age and when they transition can interplay with the personal relationship towards transition) to avoid enforcing limiting assumptions about what transition looks like.

HRT

Older people accessing HRT will have additional health considerations. For people taking oestrogen, the risk of heart disease or stroke is low, but there is an increased risk after the age of 60 (Lowe, 2004; Nudy et al, 2019). As one participant explained, "after my heart attack my GP said 'you do realise that the hormone treatment is contraindicated in this case don't you?' 'Yes.' He said 'but you're not going to stop it are you?' 'No.' 'OK fine'" (woman, aged 72). In this case, the doctor was concerned about an increased risk but still prescribed oestrogen on the basis of her informed consent. Several older participants have been put on oestrogen patches or gel instead of pills due to their physicians' belief that these delivery methods pose fewer risks (Vincent, 2018, p 155). One older woman who did not respond well to the patches described struggling to, but ultimately succeeding in, having her informed consent accepted and acquiring oestrogen pills. Another concern for older people is osteoporosis, which is directly linked to hormone levels (Vignozzi et al, 2018).

Menopause is another area where hormones and age intersect. One genderqueer man described his experience of being prescribed oestrogen for menopause:

> 'So 2016 I started menopause, I was perimenopausal before that, but I stopped bleeding in 2016 in the January and I went 23 months without bleeding and then suddenly started bleeding again. … So they gave me oestrogen, and I took it for about six weeks and then said "I don't like this, I don't like how it makes me feel". I've turned into a complete sobbing horrible wreck of a person, and I absolutely hated it. And I have to admit I did a really bad thing, and I bought some testosterone online and started taking it. And it immediately stopped my periods, and I immediately felt better. And on the oestrogen I was just bleeding constantly as well, it was just horrible. So yeah I suddenly, almost within two weeks of taking, starting [testosterone] I suddenly felt myself, I felt human again and I wasn't an emotional wreck. And my body stopped bleeding and I felt fine.' (Genderqueer man, aged 54)

For this participant, menopause reversal and the subsequent experience of oestrogen was the catalyst for them starting testosterone. Other participants also began testosterone as a result of their experiences of menopause. Older trans people may need to engage in greater self-advocacy due to clinical concern regarding potential comorbidities associated with ageing and endocrine care. This may be particularly difficult for older people who have only come out later in life and have little experience with trans communities and discourses.

Screenings

The National Health Service (NHS) offers a range of screening programmes.[2] In terms of age-based screening invitations, cervical screening is offered between the ages of 25 and 64 every five years when over the age of 49. Breast screening is offered between the ages of 50 and 70. Bowel cancer screening is offered from 60 to 74 every two years. Abdominal aortic aneurysm (AAA) is offered the year the invitee turns 65. These screening invitations rely on gender markers – patients with an 'F' marker on their records (regardless of assignment at birth, or anatomy) will be automatically invited to breast and cervical screening at the given ages. Patients with an 'M' marker will be invited for AAA, and while bowel screening also used to rely on M marker status, a process of this screening being made available to everyone started in 2021.[3] The gender markers are currently used as a proxy for the presence or absence of certain body parts and risk factors which can be a problem for anyone who does not fit into those boxes, such as a man with a cervix, or a woman without one. Specifically, it results in people not being invited for screenings they need and in some cases being invited to screenings they do not need. This can happen to someone at any age, but it was particularly prominent with the older participants as they qualify for more screenings.

Several participants reported being erroneously invited for cervical cancer screenings once they had changed their gender marker to 'F', but most were able to consent to being removed from that list when they explained to their GP that they did not require that screening. In one case, it was the GP who noticed and took responsibility to contact the patient to confirm that it was okay to remove them from the list. Doing this does not seem to have prevented anyone from continuing to receive their breast cancer screening invitations. Similarly, other participants have removed themselves from the breast cancer screening list after having top surgery while remaining on the cervical cancer screening list if relevant. In addition to removing themselves from certain screening lists, participants have also had to initiate putting themselves back on other lists, particularly for AAA and breast cancer screenings. While prostate cancer does not have a national screening programme, some transfeminine people with an 'F' marker have tried to access prostate cancer screenings with mixed success.

Breast cancer screenings were the most cited type of screening in our research and highlight the array of experiences trans people have with this type of healthcare. One man described an overall positive experience at a breast cancer screening, despite concerns he had in the lead up to the appointment:

> 'I turn up with my letter, and I'm dreading somebody making a scene like one of the nurses saying something, or somebody saying I shouldn't be there, they didn't bat an eyelid. And I think, I suspect the other people in the waiting room just thought I was sat in the wrong place ... And the woman doing the mammogram not a flicker.' (Man, aged 51)

This participant had initially gone to his GP with breast pain, which initiated an initial check as well as them being put on the regular breast cancer screening reminder list. This ease of accessing care contrasts with another participant's experience:

> 'I developed this breast abscess, and the GP's advice was go and get yourself a mammogram. So I rang Breast Test Wales to get a mammogram and was told that we don't see trans people in this service ... So I had to, my GP had to intervene ... he rang the breast consultant in the local hospital, who said "that's ridiculous, they shouldn't be discriminating like that, they should be seeing you, but I'll book you into one of my clinics because we're not going to resolve this overnight, they're not going to change the service just because I've said so". So I got booked into the local clinic to have it done in the hospital instead.' (Genderqueer man, aged 54)

This is a clear example of healthcare discrimination. This participant was not able to access the same care provision that cis women are able to access despite having the same need. Another participant described being invited for breast cancer screenings but being unsure of her need for this service:

> 'I had mammographs. I didn't go for the first two of those. I wasn't sure if I was being a fraud going, or whether they were not really meant for me, but I did go to the last one I was invited to ... And it was lovely, fine. Nobody said "oh you shouldn't be here", or anything like that.' (Non-binary woman, aged 61)

This participant's experience was ultimately positive, as were the experiences of many women in this group; however, she did miss screenings due to not feeling they were for her. While this participant was not discouraged from accessing care as the previous participant was, the absence of encouragement – such as communication from the service that it was indicated for transfeminine people with breast development following hormone access – led to healthcare avoidance. There are existing resources detailing the screening needs of trans people which these services would benefit from employing.[4] In addition, several participants suggested tracking an individual's need for various screenings, such as checkboxes to indicate the presence or absence of screening-relevant anatomy (cervix, breasts and so on). This would ensure that everyone receives the proper invitations for the body they have at that point in time.

Another reason trans people may actively avoid gendered screenings is due to dysphoria. As one participant explained:

> 'I've certainly been invited to them all my life, but my old lovely GP I told you about, he realised that I had waves of dysphoria every time he mentioned it, certain tests. So he would just mutter it under his armpit in passing because the law requires him to ask. So I wouldn't even hear. He'd just say "and it's come to that time of year again when I have to ask you. But I know you don't want that." And I'd say "you're right, I don't want it thanks". So he was respecting my wish not to be reminded of it.' (Man, aged 56)

This participant felt that this was a positive experience, because not having to have these screenings alleviated the dysphoria that accessing them would have caused. However, considering how important screening is for early detection and treatment, this is still concerning, and it highlights that the issue of proper screening provision for trans people cannot be solved by adapting administrative systems alone. Additional competency with supporting trans people experiencing dysphoria in a primary care context would be beneficial.

Hair removal

Hair removal as part of transition-related healthcare can involve general facial and body hair removal as well as targeted hair removal on a part of the body to prepare for surgery, such as hair removal on the skin graft donor site in advance of phalloplasty. The specific services provided are laser/Intense Pulsed Light (IPL) or electrolysis. Hair removal is available for trans people on the NHS, but many participants reported that the existing provision is insufficient, driving many to pay for treatment out of pocket.

For participants, hair turning white and/or grey had benefits and drawbacks. Several people pointed out that particularly white facial hair was less noticeable on them. One participant explained their decision to stop paying for private hair removal by saying "what's left is white so it's not visible anyway" (woman, aged 71). However, several participants also pointed out that laser and IPL are not effective on light hair. If the facial hair is fair, has turned white/grey or the person isn't White, electrolysis may be their only option. In those cases, the limited NHS provision is less likely to be enough, and they would have to spend more time and money out of pocket accessing private care.

Surgery later in life

As with HRT, there are additional risks for older people undergoing surgery (Turrentine et al, 2006). One participant was aware of these risks, and they were factoring into her decision-making process: "I would, I think, probably want to undertake gender reassignment or gender confirmation surgery, but I'm fully aware of age, time and the possibility that I get on the hormone treatment, and I'm happy and if that's the case, why go further with the attendant risks?" (Gender non-conforming woman, aged 58). In addition to surgical risks, some participants discussed not wanting to bother with certain surgeries because of their age:

> 'I'm undecided about the full [Sex Reassignment Surgery], I'm undecided. If I'd done this younger, then it would be an easy decision absolutely. At 63 I'm not sure. The things I would like are not things the health service will give me help for. I would dearly love to have facial feminisation, voice feminisation. Those are the things that are really important for me, but obviously they're not important to the health service. They're pretty much stuck on just sexual reassignment surgery, so I'm probably not going to get the help I require from the NHS.' (Woman, aged 62)

This woman did not feel that accessing lower surgery at her age was as important as other surgeries that are not available on the current NHS pathway. While surgery is not right for all older people, it is important that older trans people have access to good information in order to make decisions about their care and that they are able to access the care options that are best for them as individuals.

Transitioning later in life

Transitioning later in life has its own unique set of challenges. Older trans people face difficulties accessing transition-related healthcare, as discussed earlier, but participants who have transitioned later in life have described additional social barriers. Many of these participants did not know about transness early in life and, by the time they did, family and work pressures kept them in the closet. One participant describes their life in the following way:

> 'I started dressing in my mum's things from the moment I was left alone in the house, which was round about seven, eight years old; how times

change. I discovered the term transvestite when I was about 13, 14 and thought "ah OK there's other people that dress, so that must be who I am". I came out to my wife about 30 years ago now and told her I was transvestite. Didn't seem particularly right at the time, but I still couldn't really put my finger on it. … When the kids came along I went back into the closet and stayed firmly hidden away … until, where are we now, the end of 2018, beginning of 2019 when I just had a breakdown and I was positively, well, I was suicidal. It all came flooding out at that point, and I went along to the doctors and requested help.' (Woman, aged 62)

Another participant with a similar experience described what it was like to grow up not understanding that being trans was an option and feeling unsafe to explore gendered difference:

'[W]hen I was young as far as I was aware there was no such thing as transgender. There was but I wasn't aware of it. You can't be something that you don't have a concept for. … And when I was young the choice was either you're a proper boy or you're a dirty queer and we'll beat you up. And then you'll be arrested and the police will beat you up. That's probably what would have happened. And I wasn't attracted to other boys so obviously I was a proper boy because that was the only other choice. Yeah I mean gays were not at all well treated in those days. But I wasn't attracted to other boys so I must be a proper boy. So I went through most of my life that way.' (Woman, aged 71)

Even participants who did feel able to explore their identity did not come by information easily, such as this participant who sought medical support in the 1950s:

'I thought I was homosexual. So I went to see a doctor. Because there was nothing – nowadays transgender is out in the open, people talk about it. But at that time I had nothing to say "this is what you are". It was a difficult thing. I just thought I was basically a pervert, to be honest, and possibly homosexual, possibly bisexual – I was querying who I was. So that was the first time, but it didn't lead anywhere. At that time … conversion therapy and things like that, so you shoved it in the background of your mind and went on with life. And then of course it came out at odd periods, opportunities and one thing and another, and you just compartmentalised your life, your mind, so being able to continue an existence.' (Woman, aged 82)

The fear of conversion therapy prevented this person from exploring further and perhaps from transitioning earlier.

While not everyone expressed regret or negative feelings about transitioning later, some wished they had been younger and therefore at lower risk for various medical interventions. Some also feel that the changes they have experienced on hormones have been limited by their age, such as the participant who stated "If I'd done this when I was a lot younger then my facial features would have changed, they would have softened more. Given my age, the hormones they've got an uphill task" (woman, aged 68). Other participants expressed concern that not transitioning earlier meant they were not 'really trans' or were not 'trans enough', as one person explained: "I felt, one of the things I was worried about is transitioning being old. I got all tied up in this 'am I trans enough, if I'd have been really bothered I should have done this when I was 18', but when I was 18 trans men didn't exist" (man, aged 51). Of course, it was possible to transition in the early to mid-20th century, and indeed people did, but many participants lacked access to critical information and the safety and support to do so until later in life.

However, even some of those who had some level of regret around not transitioning earlier discussed feeling better prepared to do so as a result of their age. One participant who discussed having accessed oestrogen gel online said:

'I saw my GP, she wasn't willing to prescribe, but she was willing to carry out blood tests. But that didn't last very long because I realised that wasn't a sensible long-term solution to my situation. Now one advantage I had of being older, was I had resources that many people don't, and contacts as well, and knowledge.' (Gender non-conforming woman, aged 67)

Having support systems in place and knowing where to get information helped a lot of older participants in their transition. Those older participants who were retired when they transitioned explained how that was beneficial. They did not have to worry about coming out at work or taking time off for medical appointments or surgical recovery. Having children grown up and out of the house and other similar family pressures being removed were also cited as catalysts for transitioning later in life. One participant who was unable to come out earlier in life like the participants quoted previously described her experience as such:

'Historically, going through my life, I can remember crossdressing for as long as I can remember in secret ... And effectively I started getting involved into a bubble that there was no way that I could afford, if I wanted to keep my career, to be found out. So things had to be pushed and kept really secret ... Well my career in the [civil service] lasted 40 years. I carried on and worked up through grades and various bits ... going through my career in all sorts of things that I did, there was just no way I could do that.' (Woman, aged 63)

She goes on to add that marriage and children on top of the work pressures prevented her from transitioning earlier:

'We had a few children or a couple of children in reasonably quick succession after getting married and life effectively took over. And it was not really until I got into my mid 50s, I got an opportunity to retire from work, both my children were of an age where they were self-sufficient … and I found myself at home. My father had died a couple of years before who I wasn't sure about acceptance, and I found myself indoors. And other than keeping an eye out for whether anyone could see me or whatever, it was a case of I suddenly found myself, I was [name] 70 to 80 per cent of the time, and then if I knew family were coming or anything then I'd be back to my old male self just to dress up and be that. Well that carried on for a little while, probably about a year, 18 months, and then I just hit the wall of the fact that "oh God I'm trans" and in 20, as I say, it was about 2014, I had to go and see the doctor and say "look I'm trans" … as soon as I lost those pressures I was at home on my own, my children weren't around, I was living on my own. I had no money worries, I've got no commitments, I own my own house. I've got a work's pension, nobody can take my income away, all of those pressures disappeared in 2012. So once I'd got to that point I struggled on for about two years and then suddenly, no I can't cope with this anymore and yeah I'm me.' (Woman, aged 63)

Another participant described a similar situation of transitioning later in life because of the removal of certain obstacles:

'I was combining a job with of course caring for [my mum], and that took all of my time. I was doing shifts, so I had to work night shifts, and then I had to care for her during the day and so that's why I was in that position. Now, eventually of course I lost my mum and that was the only thing, because I'd retired from work so … I didn't need to work anymore, and all my caring duties were stopped, so that left me with, I didn't have any obstacles left. So that's when, it did take me three or four days of mulling it over what the consequences are, because there always is and how far-reaching they would be, so in the end I decided, well, I've done everything for everybody else, I think it's time I did something for me now, and that was the catalyst and that set me down the path.' (Woman, aged 68)

Fabbre refers to this moment as a 'dam bursting', that these people 'felt unrelenting social pressures to conform their gender identities and expressions to normative expectations throughout their lives, which often led to a desperate psychological and emotional breaking point later in life' (2017, p 482). This 'breaking point' can happen at different times and with different pressures, and while some people certainly would have transitioned earlier had they been able to do so, it is not as simple as that. Some people are happy with having transitioned later in life and have found some benefits in doing so. The key takeaway here is that if the structural and societal obstacles to living openly and accessing transition-related healthcare are removed, people may choose to transition at any age, in their own time and at their own pace.

Conclusion

Older trans people are subject to many of the same barriers to quality healthcare as the rest of the trans population, primarily long wait times to receive transition-related care. Drastically reducing these wait times is key to the health of this group. Older trans people also have unique healthcare needs, including additional challenges with hair removal and higher risks for complications from HRT and surgical interventions. These challenges should not hinder access to care, but rather providers and patients alike should be well informed, enabling the patient to make the best decision for themselves during an assessment process that is person-centred, collaborative and culturally aware of the rich diversity of trans identities. Additionally, non-transition-related care should not be ignored for older trans people. In the short term, patients and providers should be aware of what screenings and other health checks and interventions an individual needs and ensure that they receive them in a timely manner. In the long term, gender markers should be removed from medical records in favour of more accurate record keeping. Overall, older trans people are not being well served by existing healthcare systems in the UK, and sweeping systemic changes are needed to provide this population with high-quality healthcare and increased autonomy.

Notes

[1] It is important to note that people of all ages in our sample felt that they knew their own mind and expressed frustration at infantilisation from healthcare providers.
[2] While the major national screening programmes are for AAA, breast, cervical and bowel cancers, there are a range of other screenings that patients may be invited to in more specific circumstances, such as screening over the age of 12 for diabetic retinopathy for diabetic patients, or infectious disease screening in pregnant people.
[3] 'NHS screening', last reviewed 20 July 2021, Available from: https://www.nhs.uk/conditions/nhs-screening
[4] 'NHS population screening: information for trans and non-binary people', last updated 4 January 2023, Available from: https://www.gov.uk/government/publications/nhs-population-screening-information-for-transgender-people/nhs-population-screening-information-for-trans-people

References

Fabbre, V.D. (2014) 'Gender transitions in later life: the significance of time in queer aging', *Journal of Gerontological Social Work*, 57: 161–75.

Fabbre, V.D. (2017) 'Agency and social forces in the life course: the case of gender transitions in later life', *The Journals of Gerontology: Series B; Psychological Sciences and Social Sciences*, 72(3): 479–87.

Lowe, G.D.O. (2004) 'Hormone replacement therapy and cardiovascular disease: increased risks of venous thromboembolism and stroke, and no protection from coronary heart disease', *Journal of Internal Medicine*, 256(5): 361–74.

Nudy, M., Chinchilli, V.M. and Foy, A.J. (2019) 'A systematic review and meta-regression analysis to examine the "timing hypothesis" of hormone replacement therapy on mortality, coronary heart disease, and stroke', *International Journal of Cardiology Heart & Vasculature*, 22: 123–31.

Pearce, R. (2018) *Understanding Trans Health: Discourse, Power and Possibility*, Bristol: Policy Press.

Riggs, D.W., Pearce, R., Pfeffer, C.A., Hines, S., White, F. and Ruspini, E. (2019) 'Transnormativity in the psy disciplines: constructing pathology in the *Diagnostic and Statistical Manual of Mental Disorders* and *Standards of Care*', *American Psychologist*, 74(8): 912–24.

Turrentine, F.E., Wang, H., Simpson, V.B. and Jones, R.S. (2006) 'Surgical risk factors, morbidity, and mortality in elderly patients', *Journal of the American College of Surgeons*, 203(6): 865–77.

Vignozzi, L., Malavolta, N., Villa, P., Mangili, G., Migliaccio, S. and Lello, S. (2018) 'Consensus statement on the use of HRT in postmenopausal women in the management of osteoporosis by SIE, SIOMMMS and SIGO', *Journal of Endocrinological Investigation*, 42(5): 609–18.

Vincent, B. (2018) *Transgender Health: A Practitioner's Guide to Binary and Non-binary Trans Patient Care*, London: Jessica Kingsley Publishers.

Over to you

This section provides two suggested learning activities for readers that connect explicitly with the content and themes that have arisen from the two chapters in Part I. These chapters discussed what is known about older trans people's lives and care needs arising from messages from research and the significance of trans people's own perspectives and accounts on ageing and later life.

Practitioners can use these learning activities to help develop and share knowledge, skills and values that will inform the development of affirmative and person-centred support for older trans people by:

- extending your own personal and professional knowledge through relevant desktop research or practitioner enquiry;
- facilitating critical reflection and learning through active discussion in your team and service.

Educators and trainers can use these activities to:

- include trans ageing issues in the education and training of the workforce;
- guide the aim and focus of trans issues drawing on the relevant evidence provided.

Managers can use these activities to:

- embed the relevant topics, areas and learning resources into recruitment, induction, supervision, appraisal and career progression processes;
- keep a record of key activities that can be drawn upon in practice reviews or benchmarks to demonstrate how the needs of older trans people are being addressed, including the potential to demonstrate legal compliance during statutory regulatory activities.

Activity 1: Promoting trans affirmative communication for people in later life

Giving affirmation to every individual person is a unique and personal process. We use the umbrella term 'gender affirmation' to describe a range of actions that we can take to demonstrate how we are actively recognising and giving value to a person's gender identity and their desire to thrive and take joy in living, surviving and thriving as their authentic gendered selves. The following suggestions provide a guide to some of the steps you can take to support this and to stimulate discussion on your own suggestions and actions for doing so:

Suggested areas for enquiry and action	Your notes and plans
Review your service literature such as standard letters/emails/leaflets/displays to see how trans and non-binary identities are represented.	
Take active steps to display information that includes positive images of trans people in later life and their relationships.	
Check service literature and communications for gender-neutral and trans-affirmative language.	
Take steps to ensure that colleagues wear name badges with their preferred pronouns or display them in written communication, for example under your signature in emails and letters.	
Display the trans flag and wear a trans or rainbow lanyard.	
Suggest allocating gender-neutral facilities (for example, toilets and showers) in your reception or building.	

Activity 2: Equality monitoring in the access and experience of care and support for trans people in later life

It is the duty of public bodies to collect and monitor information on the range of people accessing and using their services in relation to the diversity of their characteristics where these are protected in legislation. Operationalising these requirements involves the development of questions that work as intended and that trans people feel willing and able to answer. Most importantly, feeling able to participate in equality monitoring is an area of knowledge and skill. The following tasks may be useful for all individuals and teams in working towards these:

- talk to your manager or someone with responsibility for equality data and ask for a meeting to discuss how data about gender diversity are collected, reported and monitored in your area of practice;

- where there is room for improvement, identify and raise suggestions and discuss options with senior colleagues that can help to meet standards for good practice in this area of data collection;
- work with colleagues to develop and display a short statement for trans individuals about how they can choose to share information about their gender identities and how this will be used lawfully and in a way that respects confidentiality, choice and data protection;
- with your team, develop and display a statement about your service to people in later life that commits to anti-transphobia and how individuals or groups can report transphobia to you;
- find opportunities to get feedback from individuals and the wider trans community on how this is coming across and use the feedback to inform your ongoing work in this area.

PART II

Perspectives from practice: views, attitudes and practices of healthcare and welfare professionals

3

"You know what? I'm not agreeing": older trans people's experiences of navigating, building and refusing care

Michael Toze

Introduction: writing about trans ageing

When writing about older trans people, there is a temptation to start with what a colleague once described to me as "the misery narrative". I imagine my reader to be a busy social worker, or care home manager, or perhaps a student or academic in an allied discipline who has found a few free minutes in their day to briefly read up on older trans and gender diverse people. In the face of the pressures facing such readers, I feel the pressure to capture their attention and justify the use of their time. Implicitly, I seek to defend against the accusation that this is a very small population by using terms like 'risk' or 'vulnerability' to emphasise the disproportionate harms experienced by gender diverse populations. But I am also conscious of the limitations of this narrative. It tends to flatten different experiences into a monolithic account of vulnerability, and it tends to overlook the agency and resilience of older trans people in addressing the challenges they face. In this chapter, I seek to provide a more nuanced narrative, drawing on the accounts of older trans people in the UK to explore their experiences of navigating, challenging and, at times, rejecting services available to them.

This chapter therefore seeks to explore older trans people's experiences of care from a perspective that recognises both the challenges they face and their agency and abilities in navigating those challenges across diverse life courses. It draws upon interviews undertaken as part of my doctoral thesis in 2015 and 2016 exploring the experiences of LGBT people aged 60+ in the UK within primary care. Elements of this research have been published previously (Toze et al, 2020). This analysis focuses upon the 13 participants within that study who identified as trans or transgender. Nine of the participants were trans women, two were trans men, one was non-binary and one was a transvestite who lived fluidly as both male and female. Participants were aged 60–82, predominantly retired and all lived independently in the community.

Pseudonyms have been used for most of the participants. A small number of participants emphatically did not wish to use a pseudonym, confirming this both on the day of the interview and on reviewing the transcript. For instance, one participant stated that she had been waiting for 60 years to use her preferred name, and she would never again use any other. We had a discussion about the potential implications of this, and she remained adamant that she wanted her name attached to her words. For such participants, I have used their first names in line with their wishes.

Vulnerability, robustness and resilience

My ambivalence around terms like risk or vulnerability is not because such terms are factually inaccurate. Demographic datasets have historically been poor at mapping gender diverse populations, but we do know that such populations are highly likely to report discrimination within settings such as education, employment, housing and public services (Kattari et al, 2016; Government Equalities Office, 2018). Trans people, particularly trans women, are more likely to die prematurely of causes such as suicide, homicide and poisoning (de Blok et al, 2021; Jackson et al, 2023). Older trans people are at increased risk of poor physical and mental health due to factors including disparities in diet and physical activity, poor access to healthcare and experience of discrimination (Fredriksen-Goldsen et al, 2013; Fabbre and Gaveras, 2020; Streed Jr et al, 2021). In many parts of the world, gender diversity is still implicitly or explicitly subject to state persecution: 13 countries have explicit laws criminalising 'cross-dressing', while many others use laws on issues such as vagrancy, homosexuality and public morality to target trans people (Chiam et al, 2020). Many Global North countries have introduced legal protections for trans people, but these often appear increasingly precarious. From the late 2010s onwards, several US stated have sought to restrict access to gender-affirming healthcare, predominantly targeting adolescents but including measures that also limit access to care for mature adults (Associated Press, 2023). In the UK, there have been public discussions on proposals to change the Equality Act 2010 in order to remove existing human right protections for trans people, including excluding them from health facilities that they currently access (Allegretti, 2023; Madrigal, 2023). Older trans people in many parts of the world are therefore likely to have lived through state discrimination, and even those with current protections may be concerned that these will be lost.

At the same time, against this narrative of discrimination and exclusion, my own personal and professional experience with older trans and gender diverse people has frequently been with people who were and are passionate activists and campaigners, with people involved in building communities and forming relationships, with people who are funny or argumentative or generous or irritable – and with people who are their own individual complex mix of these characteristics. I suspect many of them would not appreciate me describing them as 'vulnerable' or 'at risk', even when they are clearly experiencing substantial challenges. As one example, James, a trans man I quote later in this chapter, was in poor health and facing barriers in accessing care. He was also professionally qualified and an experienced campaigner. He spent much of the interview giving sharp critical commentary on current health policy.

Vulnerability and risk are population-level assessments, located within social factors. A population being more at risk of challenges does not mean everyone experiences those challenges, and vulnerability is not a monolithic state. Statements about vulnerability and risk are also passive formulations that conceal the agent: vulnerable to whose actions? Who is creating the risk? When I commenced this section with the statement that trans people 'are highly likely to report discrimination within settings such as education, employment, housing and public services', I was hedging the acknowledgement that such services sometimes discriminate. If older trans people are vulnerable, or at risk, or marginalised, that is a consequence of how society treats them, not an inherent aspect of who they are.

Fundamentally, trans and gender diverse people are people who, at least once in their life, have decided to express something important about who they are in a way that is likely to set them in opposition to people around them. They are also people who often have substantial experience in interacting with cisnormative systems that are not designed for them, and that frequently actively exclude them. Perhaps even more so than other demographics, it seems to me likely that a degree of resilience, resistance and sheer bloody-mindedness are frequently an important part of the picture.

The tension between identifying need and recognising strength within older gender diverse communities has been explored elsewhere. Witten (2014) titles an article 'It's not all darkness', discussing robustness (ability to resist external challenge) and resilience (ability to 'bounce back' after such challenges), concepts that are useful for mapping the reactions of older people to challenges faced. Fabbre (2014) takes a queer perspective on notions of successful ageing, presenting participants' accounts of succeeding on their own terms. Many accounts emphasise joy and personal fulfilment as components of later life transition, although these are often also balanced against other, more negative experiences (Fabbre, 2014; Willis et al, 2020; Sandberg and Holmqvist, 2023). These analyses point to a need to understand trans people's experiences of ageing on their own terms.

Another focus of academic discussion has been notions of care within trans communities. Relationships between trans communities and formal healthcare services have frequently been tense, marked by gatekeeping, exclusion and prejudice (Stone, 1991; Davy, 2011; Pearce, 2018b). Alongside this, therefore, there is also a complex ecosystem of trans peer-support networks, including support groups, magazines and the internet (FTM International, 1991; Hines, 2007; Heinz, 2016; Pearce, 2018b). Activities of such networks can include emotional support and reassurance; political and healthcare advocacy; sharing of information and experience on medical options; advice on navigating health systems; crowdfunding for private healthcare; and links to self-medication outside formal medication structures (Stone, 1991; Heinz, 2016; Pearce, 2018b; Barcelos, 2020).

The move to online spaces has made trans community networks more visible, both to prospective members and to researchers. However, while we should be cautious about stereotyping the technical skills of older adults, these online spaces do often appear to be youth oriented. For instance, studies of community and representation within sites such as YouTube report that these are typically communities focused on young adults (Eckstein, 2018; Miller, 2019). Pearce (2018a) describes one exception, Alain, a 63-year-old YouTuber, but also notes that community reactions to Alain's video often focused upon his apparent youthfulness. While the reported discussion is clearly supportive, it seems to be framed around Alain as an exception within a space that is not normally occupied by over-60s.

Pearce (2018a) highlights the complexity of trans temporalities: trans people discuss age in terms of both chronological age and key markers of life as a trans person, such as coming out or accessing medical care. As such, an 80-year-old who transitioned 50 years ago and an 80-year-old transitioning now both are and are not the same age: while both may have been born in the same year, the experiences of transitioning in the 1970s and of transitioning in the 2020s are in many respects different. That is not to say chronological age is irrelevant: the 80-year-old who is transitioning now is also likely to have different experiences from a 20-year-old who is transitioning. Understanding trans experiences through online spaces that tend to cater for young adults who are early in their transition is therefore likely to overlook important dimensions of experience for those who are 'older' in either or both ways of counting: those who are chronologically older, and those who have been navigating life as a trans person for many years. Both groups may have different experiences of challenges, and of the strategies and robustness required to navigate those challenges.

Transition pathways and possibilities

Witten (2009) distinguishes between trans people who came out as trans in early life and then aged, and those who transitioned when they were already in later life. Most of the trans people I spoke to described the latter trajectory, although one participant, James, had transitioned in his teenage years. Most participants also emphasised that later life transition would not have been their choice. Rather, it was because transition had been impossible or unthinkable in their past:

> 'I'd love to have done it years ago. Love to. I mean my first experience, or my first memory was when I was about seven years of age. My dad caught me. Never said a word. In those days, in about – when would that have been? About 1961, '62 – you just didn't talk about stuff like that. You know, it just wasn't done. Would have been seen as "you dirty so and so", it was just, y'know. It wasn't done.' (Laura, trans woman)

The concept of trans 'possibility models', articulated by the actress Laverne Cox, highlights that seeing representations and examples of other trans people living their lives often makes it easier for trans people to see 'coming out' as a viable possibility (Pearce et al, 2019). Several participants gave accounts that resonated with this concept, with very distinct memories of moments when possibilities of being trans opened up for them.

Like Laura, Sally described an initial time of isolation, in which gender diversity was taboo:

> 'At that stage, you know the internet didn't exist … So far as I was aware I was the only transvestite in the world. I'd not seen any transvestite magazines or books about them, and I hadn't met another one. I only knew the word because I'd seen it in the dictionary, and I knew it didn't suit me cos it said there at the end that a transvestite was a pervert.' (Sally, transvestite)

A 'transformation moment' for Sally came from a light entertainment radio show:

> 'This reporter said that she was with a group of people who'd all got something in common and they were just on a coach and they were going out to visit a vineyard somewhere in the south of Britain and they were all on holiday together. And she says what they've got together in common is they're all transvestites. And I couldn't believe – this was teatime on Radio 4 and as far as I knew transvestites were perverts and here was the BBC talking about them … It was a transformation moment.' (Sally, transvestite)

Another participant described realising he was a trans man in his 70s through research for a creative writing group:

'Somebody challenged me to write a gay story, and so I started researching ... As far as my son was concerned, I was wasting me time, but as far as I was concerned it was filling in the gaps, and I was teaching myself what I was, what I am.' (Joe, trans man)

However, he suggested that for some older trans people, fear might continue to inhibit the perceived possibility of living life as a trans person:

Joe: This is the problem with the over-60s, they're afraid to say even to a friend, to say I'm a transgender male or a transgender woman.
MT: Why do you think people are afraid?
Joe: If they read the kind of stories that I read on the internet about the horrors that gay people and transgendered people have, being attacked, criticised and brutalised, maybe it's that that's in their minds eye. "Ooh I'm, I'm over 60, I couldn't do that. Couldn't do that, so button your lip." (Joe, trans man)

Amy had identified a route to gender-affirming care while she was a young adult. However, the potential social consequences had seemed insurmountable, and she had ultimately decided not to proceed at that time:

'I did at that time find a GP who was willing to prescribe hormones and so on, but that was in 1971. However, I wanted a family, I wanted a career, and it seemed like it was just too much to contemplate trying to do that as essentially I would be a transgender person who was lesbian, and let's face it there wasn't exactly a great deal of either understanding or tolerance for those kinds of things in the 1970s.' (Amy, trans woman)

These accounts reflect just some of the diversity that may exist within older trans people's life stories. Transitioning in later life may be perceived by others as being a change in identity. However, older trans people may be more likely to describe it as discovering concepts and a community that allow for better self-understanding and self-expression. Many accounts emphasised the extent that social context could inhibit someone's ability to live life as a trans person. Changes to that social context, the discovery of community and self-realisation, were factors that made life as a trans person seem more possible and provided individuals with the strength, resilience and self-determination to live as they chose.

Experiences of formal health services

Eleven of the 13 participants in this study had taken medical steps towards transition. In the UK, medical transition is available through the National

Health Service (NHS), requiring a general practitioner to refer a patient to a specialist gender clinic. Most participants indicated that their general practitioner was supportive, if not necessarily knowledgeable. However, as outlined by Callahan et al in the previous chapter, many participants highlighted barriers to accessing NHS care, particularly around waiting times and lack of flexibility to individual needs, often necessitating alternative routes to care.

Amy had commenced her transition in France and then relocated to the UK. The NHS gender clinic and the commissioning body disagreed over how to manage the continuation of her hormone medication while she was waiting for a UK appointment, with both agreeing she should continue her medicine but neither accepting responsibility for prescribing. As a consequence, Amy was travelling to France to access prescriptions there:

'[The gender clinic] sent [my GP] a letter stating that I was on hormones and anti-androgens and that they should take over the medication on an interim basis ... What I got back of course was some letter from the clinical care group saying no way, it was nothing to do with them it was down to [the gender clinic] ... So as far as I'm concerned it was bloody nonsense, they were just kind of passing the buck ... So I went back to France last month, and I actually already had an appointment from the previous year with the endocrinologist so I went back to see him.' (Amy, trans woman)

Other participants reported historically restrictive clinical protocols within the NHS gender clinics, with factors such as age and body type sometimes used to decline care. Helen had decided to not even try to use NHS services: "I didn't actually go through the NHS for my treatment. I was in my 50s, overweight, too tall, smoked, so all those were contra indicators for NHS treatment. So I had an insurance policy coming up for maturity so I borrowed off that to fund my surgery" (Helen, trans woman).

Frankie had accessed NHS services but found that standardised pathways for chest surgery did not address their needs as a non-binary trans masculine person with a larger build. They were encouraged to agree to a total mastectomy that they did not want and ultimately opted out of a surgery referral altogether:

'I was talking about breast surgery, and I said ... I don't have an identity that's 100 per cent male, and in any case a male of my age and build isn't going to have a dead flat chest cos it just doesn't work like that ... I said I'd like to go smaller cos I get a lot of scarring and soreness under here and I used to bind at the time more often. And they said: "Oh, we can't do that" ... They said: "We can only refer you for a mastectomy, you know, if you agree to a total mastectomy" and all that. And I eventually said: "You know what? I'm not agreeing."' (Frankie, non-binary person)

At the time Sophie decided to transition, she did not feel emotionally ready to approach her GP. Instead, she commenced self-medicating by buying medicine online: "I didn't approach my GP at the time. I probably wasn't in the right place emotionally and mentally to do that. So what I did was I started self-medding. I know it's not what you should do but I was doing it at the time" (Sophie, trans woman).

Accessing care outside NHS pathways appears to be common among older trans people. Bouman et al (2016) report that half of older trans women patients at one NHS gender clinic had already accessed hormone medication elsewhere, through routes such as private care or self-medication. Those who had already accessed care also tended to have better psychological wellbeing, somewhat bringing into question whether lengthy care pathways are fit for purpose. However, accessing medication outside NHS pathways may also have disadvantages, for example with regard to continuity of care, and the potential risks of counterfeit medications when self-medicating.

Several participants in this study were retired from professional careers and commented that they were fortunate that their financial status made it easier for them to find alternative sources of care. However, Elizabeth, who was unable to work, highlighted the financial and logistical burdens she faced in self-medicating while waiting for a gender clinic appointment:

'I had to research it all on the internet, it took me months. First of all I had to find out, and mostly off American websites and then get the English equivalent which isn't easy cos they often don't want to give you the information. Then when you do find a chemist warehouse that is willing to sell you them off prescription the prices are exorbitant, I mean through the roof silly. At the moment with my income support I'm spending about £188 a month plus the customs and excise fee plus the postal fee and the only way I've found round that … is to order everything separate so it comes in little packets and can travel through the airmail … but it's took me a year to find that out so you know initially it was costing us £230, £240 a month. Bloody killed us.' (Elizabeth, trans woman)

Participants who were accessing NHS care also sometimes highlighted uncertainty and lack of clarity in their care. James had transitioned in his teenage years and had long since been discharged from specialist services. This led to disagreement over who could authorise changes to his testosterone medication when he experienced polycythaemia, a known side effect that can often be aided by moving to other formulations:

> 'I think for a while I had a hotline to a special department within the primary care trust cos of my hormones. And they had, they put a block and so I went to the GP and said "Well, I don't know if I'm allowed to move to cream, I want to." "But I don't know if I can because it's not the same brand as what you've had before." That was the excuse right … it happened several times because of my polycythaemia.' (James, trans man)

Eleanor was extremely happy with the care she received locally. She had considered moving closer to her daughter but decided not to, in part because moving might disrupt her care:

> 'That was definitely one of the factors. Well, do I really – is it sensible to move down there when all the support I'm getting is here and everything is so very quick and smooth and I don't have any problems? Down there I've got to start all over again.' (Eleanor, trans woman)

Participants' experience of formal health services was often that processes were slow, inflexible and did not always meet their needs. While participants often also described good experiences, particularly with GPs, there was often a sense that this could not be taken for granted.

Participants demonstrated knowledge, agency and resilience in working around the system and finding alternative options to access care in the face of setbacks. But this was also often burdensome, incurring extra costs, time or restricting other options such as geographic mobility. Some of the 'work around' arrangements described – travelling to France for prescriptions, purchasing medication online or contacting a particular NHS department for support – were dependent on a combination of personal determination and identifying sympathetic professionals, as well as being eased by health literacy and financial resources. Such arrangements were potentially precarious and not necessarily sustainable if the individual became more dependent on assistance from others or if health service personnel changed.

Experiences of community, campaigning and care

Participants for this study were recruited through community sector networks and 'snowballing'. Perhaps as a consequence, most belonged to trans and LGBTQ+ groups. Some had a long history of involvement in organisations campaigning on issues related to trans healthcare and social inclusion. James had been involved in both developing and challenging national trans health guidelines, describing specific instances where he was certain he had successfully influenced decision making within the NHS and other bodies. James and I agreed that I would not directly quote his accounts of these meetings, due to the difficulty in anonymisation.

Helen similarly had a long history of working with advocacy groups but pointed to some of the challenges. At one stage, she reflected on the nature of trans community and community work:

> 'If you can get the trans community to work as one group [laughs] you're a better person than I am. It is such a fragmented community, and some people would challenge whether there is actually a community at all. I think there is, if you look at the definition, but so many people have slightly different viewpoints on approaches and then set up their own little organisations to promote their specific approach. And trying to get them to work together. I mean we did try and set up [a trans umbrella organisation], gosh, it must be getting on for eight, nine years ago now. ... But trying to get people to, sort of work together wasn't easy and when I left, resigned as Chair of one of the charities, and then stopped attending one of the ... meetings it seemed to dissipate.' (Helen, trans woman)

Other people's experiences of groups focused on individual support. Mirroring the observation that many older trans people had grown up believing that being trans was shameful, Anne highlighted the benefits of a group in helping individuals address their fears and internalised stigma:

> 'A group is very helpful for people starting out or people who do not know within themselves what they are doing. They feel very nervous about it, they feel it's some kind of dreadful perversion and they'll be perhaps divorced, popped in a nuthouse, certified, have people laughing at them. There's a whole range of fears, but the only way to overcome them is by learning and time.' (Anne, trans woman)

Caroline described being involved in a mixture of both individual support and political advocacy for trans people and their loved ones. Much of this work was done in conjunction with her wife:

> 'After the initial shock and grief for [my wife] she has been extremely supportive of me and ... has got involved to the point where she is also supporting trans people and SOFFAs [Significant Others, Family, Friends and Allies] so we're really quite a combined unit. For a considerable number of years I was on the board of trustees for [a charity] ... and in fact I am still the Chair but we're, we're just in the

process of closing the charity down unfortunately because we couldn't get any more funding. So we've been quite involved in in the scene in all sorts of ways.' (Caroline, trans woman)

Caroline's and Helen's accounts point to the fragility and precarity of relatively small networks that are potentially vulnerable to closure due to lack of funding or key volunteers leaving.

Precarity and fragmentation in the sector also potentially created issues when organisations tried to signpost trans people to voluntary sector support. Elizabeth showed me a list of support groups that had been given to her by the NHS but was scathing about it. Most of the groups were not relevant. In one case, the website had been hacked, resulting in her computer getting a virus:

> 'It's a list of supposed support groups. You'll find there's one on there that destroyed a 1,000-pound laptop because it was virused that badly when I went on it, it destroyed it. So none of those on there are of any relevance whatsoever for a male to female transgender, absolutely none.' (Elizabeth, trans woman)

Elizabeth had ultimately identified for herself a more appropriate support group, although it was some distance away. It seems likely that the problems in the list were linked to the diversity and fluidity in the trans voluntary sector. Weblinks may become unsafe when a small charity folds and does not renew its domain name. It may not be immediately obvious to someone unfamiliar with the trans community that a particular support group is (for instance) focused upon those who do not wish to make a permanent transition or on younger trans men and hence not appropriate for an older trans woman. Simply creating a list of voluntary groups may therefore not be helpful if time is not taken to check they are up to date and to tailor signposting for individual needs.

Some participants were less sure about wanting to join trans groups at all. Eleanor was clearly ambivalent on the subject:

> 'I'm not a great one for leaping into sort of social things like that unless I feel comfortable. I mean I'll do things like, you know motor sport, I join motor clubs, sailing, yeah, but something like that I'll, I – no, I'd rather just live life normally, without feeling that I've got to join a bunch of people all of whom are like me. And I just, I just never sort of … I think it would be nice to sort of meet up with somebody like me on a social group level, not to go to a social meeting with a group of people like me because … In a lot of cases my background is rather different because I was brought up overseas.' (Eleanor, trans woman)

There are multiple broken sentences in Eleanor's account here, perhaps indicating that she was struggling to articulate her exact feelings on the issue. Overall, it seemed that Eleanor was potentially interested in meeting peers but concerned that a trans-focused group might not actually help her meet people she would feel she had something in common with. She indicated that she would ideally prefer to meet another trans woman within the networks she already belonged to rather than seeking out trans groups.

Overall, most participants described trans community groups as offering benefits, both for organising and campaigning and for finding peer support. These groups potentially increased members' ability to navigate challenges and indeed campaign for improvements. However, many of their answers also pointed to difficulties within the sector. These often related to the structural issues involved in relatively small, unfunded groups covering large geographic areas and diverse populations. In the UK LGBT voluntary sector as a whole, the majority of organisations are 'micro' or 'small', experiencing funding challenges due to austerity and, more recently, COVID-19 (Colgan et al, 2014; Consortium, 2020). It is likely that these issues are amplified for groups appropriate for older trans people, who represent an even smaller sub-set of the population. While professionals and public services might hope to draw on the voluntary sector to help them support trans older people, the capacity of such groups may be limited. Effective community building and partnership between professionals and community groups, along with appropriate resourcing, is therefore important in order to utilise the experience and skills that exist in trans groups without overburdening small organisations and their volunteers.

Conclusion

In this chapter, I have sought to explore the complex ways in which older trans people may navigate transition, community, health and care. For many of the people I spoke to, existing services were not well suited to their needs and were characterised by delays and inflexibility. Community and voluntary sector organisations provided a potential alternative but often themselves lacked resilience, being small and volunteer dependent. Importantly, many participants were directly involved in running such organisations rather than passively receiving support.

Despite the challenges, participants clearly articulated agency and skill in navigating life as an older trans person and personal sources of resilience and robustness. Several of them had taken leadership roles within campaigning or community groups. Others had taken action to challenge or to work around health systems that were not meeting their needs. Most also emphasised the resources they were drawing on, whether those were financial resources, personal skills and knowledge, or support networks. Even for those who clearly faced substantial challenges, their accounts generally emphasised the ways in which they were active in responding to those difficulties, demonstrating robustness, resilience and agency in navigating barriers and recovering from challenges.

For those working with older trans people, there is a need to recognise the importance of these past life experiences in how people may access services and care later in life. Older trans people may be justifiably cynical about whether they expect mainstream services to be thoughtful and considerate to their needs and have developed their own, alternative routes to get needs met. Community groups may be an important source of support but are also often small, precarious and subject to volunteer 'churn'. This may offer scope for community-building work between professionals and the voluntary sector in order to build effective partnerships and share expertise, creating resilience within trans communities.

Summary learning points

- Older trans people have very diverse life experiences. Those who 'come out' as trans later in life may have previous experience of barriers or challenges that made it impossible for them to do so sooner.
- Older trans people are likely to have previously experienced public services that are poorly configured to their needs. They may have experience of challenging services, or of needing to be independent in managing their own care. This may influence expectations and interactions with services later in life.
- Building links with the voluntary and community sector can be beneficial. However, there may be relatively few groups with experience in supporting trans older people, and they will often be small, financially precarious and volunteer-run. It may be useful for practitioners to consider longer-term support for community development.

References

Allegretti, A. (2023) 'What would changing the Equality Act mean for trans people and single-sex spaces?', *The Guardian*, Available from: https://www.theguardian.com/law/2023/apr/05/what-would-changing-the-equality-act-mean-for-trans-people-and-single-sex-spaces

Associated Press (2023) 'Trans adults in Florida "blindsided" that new law also limits their access to health care', NBC News, Available from: https://www.nbcnews.com/nbc-out/out-news/trans-adults-florida-blindsided-new-law-also-limits-access-health-care-rcna87723

Barcelos, C.A. (2020) 'Go fund inequality: the politics of crowdfunding transgender medical care', *Critical Public Health*, 30(3): 330–39.

Bouman, W.P., Claes, L., Marshall, E., Pinner, G.T., Longworth, J., Maddox, V. et al (2016) 'Sociodemographic variables, clinical features, and the role of preassessment cross-sex hormones in older trans people', *The Journal of Sexual Medicine*, 13(4): 711–19.

Chiam, Z., Duffy, S., Gil, M.G., Goodwin, L. and Patel, N.T.M. (2020) 'Trans legal mapping report 2019', Geneva: ILGA, Available from: https://ilga.org/downloads/ILGA_World_Trans_Legal_Mapping_Report_2019_EN.pdf

Colgan, F., Hunter, C. and McKearney, A. (2014) '"Staying alive": the impact of "austerity cuts" on the LGBT voluntary and community sector (VCS) in England and Wales', London: Trades Union Congress, Available from: https://www.tuc.org.uk/sites/default/files/StayingAlive.pdf

Consortium (2020) 'An insight into the effect of COVID-19 on the LGBT+ sector in the UK', Exeter: Consortium, Available from: https://www.consortium.lgbt/wp-content/uploads/2019/07/The-Impact-of-CV19-on-LGBT-Organisations.pdf

Davy, Z. (2011) *Recognising Transsexuals: Personal, Political and Medicolegal Embodiment*, Farnham: Ashgate.

De Blok, C.J., Wiepjes, C.M., Van Velzen, D.M., Staphorsius, A.S., Nota, N.M., Gooren, L.J.G. et al (2021) 'Mortality trends over five decades in adult transgender people receiving hormone treatment: a report from the Amsterdam cohort of gender dysphoria', *The Lancet Diabetes & Endocrinology*, 9(10): 663–70.

Eckstein, A.J. (2018) 'Out of sync: complex temporality in transgender men's YouTube transition channels', *QED: A Journal in GLBTQ Worldmaking*, 5(1): 24–47.

Fabbre, V.D. (2014) 'Gender transitions in later life: a queer perspective on successful aging', *The Gerontologist*, 55(1): 144–53.

Fabbre, V.D. and Gaveras, E. (2020) 'The manifestation of multilevel stigma in the lived experiences of transgender and gender nonconforming older adults', *American Journal of Orthopsychiatry*, 90(3): 350–60.

Fredriksen-Goldsen, K.I., Cook-Daniels, L., Kim, H.-J., Erosheva, E.A., Emlet, C.A., Hoy-Ellis, C.P. et al (2013) 'Physical and mental health of transgender older adults: an at-risk and underserved population', *The Gerontologist*, 54(3): 488–500.

FTM International (1991) 'FTM newsletter #18', California: FTM International, Available from: https://www.digitaltransgenderarchive.net/files/nk322d54j

Government Equalities Office (2018) 'National LGBT survey: research report', London, Available from: https://www.gov.uk/government/publications/national-lgbt-survey-summary-report

Heinz, M. (2016) *Entering Transmasculinity: The Inevitability of Discourse*, Bristol: Intellect.

Hines, S. (2007) 'Transgendering care: practices of care within transgender communities', *Critical Social Policy*, 27(4): 462–86.

Jackson, S.S., Brown, J., Pfeiffer, R.M., Shrewsbury, D., O'Callaghan, S., Berner, A.M. et al (2023) 'Analysis of mortality among transgender and gender diverse adults in England', *JAMA Network Open*, 6(1): e2253687–e2253687, Available from: https://doi.org/10.1001/jamanetworkopen.2022.53687

Kattari, S.K., Whitfield, D.L., Walls, N.E., Langenderfer-Magruder, L. and Ramos, D. (2016) 'Policing gender through housing and employment discrimination: comparison of discrimination experiences of transgender and cisgender LGBQ individuals', *Journal of the Society for Social Work and Research*, 7(3): 427–47.

Madrigal, V. (2023) 'United Nations independent expert on protection against violence and discrimination based on sexual orientation and gender identity: country visit to the United Kingdom of Great Britain and Northern Ireland (24 April–5 May 2023); end of mission statement', Geneva: United Nations, Available from: https://www.ohchr.org/sites/default/files/documents/issues/sexualorientation/statements/eom-statement-UK-IE-SOGI-2023-05-10.pdf

Miller, J.F. (2019) 'YouTube as a site of counternarratives to transnormativity', *Journal of Homosexuality*, 66(6): 815–37.

Pearce, R. (2018a) 'Trans temporalities and non-linear ageing', in A. King, K. Almack, Y.-T. Suen and S. Westwood (eds) *Older Lesbian, Gay, Bisexual and Trans People: Minding the Knowledge Gaps*, London: Routledge, pp 61–74.

Pearce, R. (2018b) *Understanding Trans Health: Discourse, Power and Possibility*, Bristol: Policy Press.

Pearce, R., Gupta, K. and Moon, I. (2019) 'Introduction: the many-voiced monster; collective determination and the emergence of trans', in R. Pearce, I. Moon, K. Gupta and D.L. Steinberg (eds) *The Emergence of Trans: Cultures, Politics and Everyday Lives*, London: Routledge, pp 1–12.

Sandberg, L.J. and Holmqvist, S. (2023) '"Daring to be true and to shine brightly in the time that remains": imagining transgender ageing in Fredrik Ekelund's Q', *NORA: Nordic Journal of Feminist and Gender Research*, 31(3): 292–305.

Stone, S. (1991) 'The empire strikes back: a posttranssexual manifesto', in J. Epstein and K. Straub (eds) *Body Guards: The Cultural Politics of Gender Ambiguity*, New York: Routledge, pp 280–304.

Streed Jr, C.G., Beach, L.B., Caceres, B.A., Dowshen, N.L., Moreau, K.L., Mukherjee, M. et al (2021) 'Assessing and addressing cardiovascular health in people who are transgender and gender diverse: a scientific statement from the American Heart Association', *Circulation*, 144(6): e136–e148.

Toze, M., Fish, J., Hafford-Letchfield, T. and Almack, K. (2020) 'Applying a capabilities approach to understanding older LGBT people's disclosures of identity in community primary care', *International Journal of Environmental Research and Public Health*, 17(20): 7614–32.

Willis, P., Raithby, M., Dobbs, C., Evans, E. and Bishop, J.-A. (2020) '"I'm going to live my life for me": trans ageing, care, and older trans and gender non-conforming adults' expectations of and concerns for later life', *Ageing & Society*, 41(12): 2792–813.

Witten, T.M. (2009) 'Graceful exits: intersection of aging, transgender identities, and the family/community', *Journal of GLBT Family Studies*, 5(1–2): 35–61.

Witten, T.M. (2014) 'It's not all darkness: robustness, resilience, and successful transgender aging', *LGBT Health*, 1(1): 24–33.

4

Not in the family: trans people's experiences of family relationships and the implications for support in later life

Trish Hafford-Letchfield, Christine Cocker, Keira McCormack and Rebecca Manning

Introduction

This chapter looks more closely at the challenges and opportunities that trans people face when accessing family and social support in later life. Social support is often cited as an important factor contributing to subjective wellbeing as one gets older (Diener and Seligman, 2002), and earlier chapters have already discussed some of the cumulative life experiences for trans people which may impact on access to the health and social care services they may use to support themselves in later life. In some global regions, there is a general presumption that an ageing population will give rise to an increased need for health and social care services. This is a complex picture (Health Foundation, 2021), and the demand for care will also be influenced by the availability of unpaid and informal care provided by family and friends. The picture for trans people in later life may however be more complex in terms of who is best placed to support them and the choices they have available. In Chapter 2, Callahan and colleagues articulate some of the proactive choices and responses to care barriers experienced when engaging with services that have historically not welcomed them. In Chapter 3, Toze highlighted the health and social care network alternatives created by and for trans people but which are often small and fragile and vulnerable to macro-economic and political influences. To be able to plan future service delivery effectively, policy makers will need to understand how any changes in population structure will impact overall demand; other authors in this book have discussed some of the barriers and necessary changes required to achieve this in relation to the ageing trans population. A social constructionist approach can also help us to critically examine discourses present within the wider cultural environment about ageing, families and caring and to challenge normative understandings about what a family is, to appreciate what might be different, similar or unique for older trans people.

This chapter draws on some of the themes from the authors' findings in relation to a systematic review on the international literature on what is known about trans parenting (Hafford-Letchfield et al, 2019). This review established that there were very limited findings on grandparenting and parenting later in the life course, as well as where a parent is trans, how the dynamics of family life impacted on their subsequent life course experiences. We summarise the relative themes from this body of literature to examine the potential implications for accessing and developing support in later life particularly where individual parenting rights have been transgressed and subsequent inequalities interact with planning for future care. We then draw on some unreported empirical data from a subsequent UK study of professional perspectives on trans parenting (Hafford-Letchfield et al, 2021). This includes contributions from one trans participant who shared their reflections on their own family life and growing older, and one medical professional working with a trans older person who had been referred to the gender identity clinic (GIC). Combined with other literature sources, we aim to summarise key messages for professional practice with trans people in later life in response to these findings.

What is known about trans parenting through the life course?

There is limited data on family and other informal support networks for older trans people in the UK, but we know that many trans people are parents (Riggs et al, 2016; Charter et al, 2023). In the UK, Bouman et al (2016) report that of the trans women aged 50+ newly referred to a UK gender identity clinic, 63 per cent had children and 27 per cent were currently married or in a civil partnership. The UK Government Equalities Office LGBT survey (Government Equalities Office, 2018) received responses from around 900 trans people over the age of 55 but did not capture their parental status. The survey did however report that 44 per cent of trans people aged 55–64 and 39 per cent of those aged 65+ were married, in a civil partnership or cohabiting with a partner (see Toze et al, 2023a). Other international studies have reported up to 50 per cent of trans people being parents (Grant et al, 2011); and for those who affirm their gender later in life, up to 80 per cent are parents (Pyne, 2015; Stotzer, 2014). In another study, non-representative estimates indicate that 25 to 50 per cent of transgender people are parents (Carone et al, 2021). These figures are likely underestimates, as there are difficulties in collecting comprehensive demographic information about this group, because few national surveys ask about gender identity (Herman, 2014; see also Chapter 1 by Kneale et al). Yet very little is known about their demographic characteristics and health outcomes, particularly their experiences of parenting in later life, including being a grandparent (Hafford-Letchfield et al, 2019). Even in the most supportive families, affirming gender identity can be alternatively experienced as a significant loss for other individuals within family relationships. There is little research on how the trans individual experiences any negotiation or re-establishment of family relationships at the time, as well as how they balance these with their own needs and journey throughout the life course (Haines et al, 2014). The literature also acknowledges that some trans people themselves experience loss because they were not able to achieve being a parent earlier in their life course. This may be due to lack of support from their family in having a family or having experienced lack of choice or access to affirming medical interventions (von Doussa Power and Riggs, 2015) or being excluded from alternative routes to becoming a parent or carer such as through adoption and fostering (Cocker, 2022).

Our own systematic review sought to evaluate existing findings from empirical research on trans parenting/grandparenting to understand how trans people negotiate their relationships with their partners, co-parents and children following transition and to consider the implications for professional practice with trans people in relation to how best to support them with their family caring roles or changes in those roles in later life. Most studies in this review depended on small samples: the range for qualitative studies (using interviews and focus groups) was between three and 50 individuals, and the range for quantitative studies (namely online surveys) was from 14 to 6,456 respondents, although most surveys involved fewer than 100 people. These samples reflect the challenges in researching the topic and population, particularly in relation to achieving diverse samples to illustrate ageing, cultural or indigenous parenting and family practices. Many featured in-depth case studies, using individual biographies to illustrate experiences and practices of partnering and parenting in families where a parent is trans (see Hines, 2006). Myriad challenges were documented within the literature in relation to the impact of being a trans parent on children, relationships with partners, co-parents and wider families within a transphobic and discriminatory society. As stated earlier, we found no studies on grandparents and grandchildren. Being on a journey to affirm one's gender identity has been described as a multifaceted process that may begin with the individual recognising, acknowledging and accepting, which can happen in stages over time (Charter et al, 2023) and when an individual may already be a parent or grandparent. We know that concealment of identity or self-limitation of gender expression may also contribute to minority stress, internalised prejudice and depression within older trans populations (Toze et al, 2023b).

More broadly, the literature documents considerable turmoil in families, exacerbated by disapproval and stigmatisation from outside the immediate family, from other relatives and their wider social, educational and work circles (Toyoshima and Nakahara, 2021; Freeman et al, 2002). Family conflict was a significant risk factor affecting children, especially due to the response and support from a partner or co-parent, which could be more negatively impactful than their parent being trans (White and Ettner, 2004). Concerns about the trans person's influence on children can be seen by co-parents as outweighing their concerns about the impact of reducing or even ceasing contact between the child and their trans parent. This can result in the loss of relationships over years. For the trans parent, careful management of their visibility in the community where their parenting is under intense scrutiny, from ex partners, the court system and from the wider community (Pyne et al, 2015) was further complicated by judicial adversarial processes and lack of therapeutic support for those involved (Grant et al, 2011). Trans parents found it difficult to reach out for help for fear of having the care of their children brought into question (Pyne et al, 2015; Riggs et al, 2016). Parents were also found to move away from friends or family to escape these difficulties (McNeil et al, 2012).

In terms of the life course, some studies documented much longer-term negative outcomes for trans parents, including homelessness, unemployment, increased psychological vulnerability and suicide attempts. Participants learned that there is no point in help seeking due to unsupported services resulting in both lack of confidence and skills in doing so and/or keeping a low profile. These experiences and circumstances have been shown to affect trans parents' economic situation, where they were more likely to be living in poverty or near poverty (Barnes et al, 2006; Pyne, 2015). For example, for older people family breakdown may adversely affect their subsequent pensions and ability to accumulate income and other resources for later life. It is therefore logical, in the absence of any empirical literature, to conclude that for trans people these experiences can subsequently affect both their emotional and material resources (including their pensions) in later life, which in turn affect their health and wellbeing.

More positively, findings from the review also highlighted how trans parents were very concerned about the wellbeing of their children and sought to protect them from the stigma and discrimination they faced themselves (Haines et al, 2014). There were examples of strong reciprocal climates of emotional and practical care demonstrated between parents and their children (Hines, 2006). Understanding these histories and trajectories is important for any assessment undertaken with trans people in later life. Wider family acceptance and support at any time of life has been found to be a protective factor by providing a safety net, better health outcomes and higher levels of social and economic security (Toyoshima and Nakahara, 2021; Cosby and Berry-Edwards, 2022). Acceptance and assistance from wider families promoted a strong sense of coherence and positive family functioning for trans parents. It is important for practitioners and professionals not to make assumptions about trans older people and to take time to explore an individual's narratives about family and alternative support networks and find ways of evaluating any protective factors (Veldorale-Griffin and Darling, 2016). Acceptance by families of trans lives is associated with greater self-esteem and life satisfaction, even in the face of pervasive mistreatment and discrimination outside of the home (Valdorale-Griffin, 2014: Riggs et al, 2016). Affirmation and acceptance also encompasses the notion that older people make a valuable contribution to society and the economy, including through continued employment, informal care for grandchildren and other relatives, and volunteering. As already known in relation to the reliance and significance of their 'families of choice' in wider LGBQ populations (Donovan et al, 2001), trans individuals have also been shown to have more close friends than family members they could confide in and in many circumstances would be more likely to contact friends than partners or family members for urgent support (McNeil et al, 2012).

A study of trans parenting which included a few older participants (Charter et al, 2023) revealed that trans parents affirming their gender identity in later life found it more of a gradual reveal. One 60-year-old person in this study, with three adult children and two grandchildren, found that they felt supported to come out in their own time and had the opportunities to talk to their adult children who already understood trans identities. Another participant in their 50s talked about being more present, more relaxed and much happier as a parent following transition; both noted that their adult children were already aware that something was going on for them, and this theme of family acceptance and support was crucial to feeling happier in later life.

Insights from trans parents' experiences

We now move on to share some insights regarding older trans individuals from an empirical study that explored the practices and meaning of 'parenting' and 'caring' for care professionals in families with parents with diverse gender identities in the UK. We draw on selected unreported data from a qualitative study that aimed to capture a snapshot of the current state of practice knowledge and perceived practice challenges (Hafford-Letchfield et al, 2021). These were based on detailed consultations with 25 relevant stakeholders in the proxy roles identified from the systematic review of what is known about trans parenting from the research evidence discussed earlier. One of the informants was a medical professional working within a UK GIC and the other was an older parent with adult children and grandchildren, who also volunteers within a national charity organisation that supports LGBTQ+ people. These (anonymised) circumstances provide two potential scenarios faced by older trans people that illustrate the complexities and dilemmas that can occur for parents and the choices they are faced with.

Scenario 1

Martha (not her real name) is a medical doctor who works within a multidisciplinary team which comprises a UK regional GIC and offered the following experience when participating in a focus group with the team:

> 'I work with a trans woman who has felt a lot of social pressure not to transition. She is in a relationship and has split from her wife. She hasn't undertaken a social gender transition but started taking hormones and is really positive about that, that was a really good experience. She has two daughters, one of whom was supportive suggesting that they go out together to spaces where her parent can feel comfortable. However, her other daughter has a younger child, who is maybe five or something like that and when she found out about, who she views as her father taking hormone treatment, she essentially said, "you can't see your grandchild. You can't see your grandchild until you stop this nonsense." And he's stopped, not even transitioning, he stopped hormone treatment and that's what this person did and that's put them in a real bind. For other medical reasons, they don't have gonads, that has put them in a real bind, because they don't want to take testosterone but then from an emotional and social perspective, they feel unable to take oestrogens because they are being cut off from people that they love. And that, you know is an impossible situation for them. They asked to be discharged [from the GID clinic], they've come back, they are coming back at the moment, because I think that's been, I don't know, but I imagine that's created some intolerable pain for them. It's the adult child not being able to accept that their parent is gender diverse and being really resistant to the idea that the person that they viewed as their dad, might not have been that person's authentic self and being able to accept it.'

Scenario 2

Martinez (not her real name), a White British trans woman who is aged 67 years, reflected on her married life, having realised she wanted to be female from an early age but was assigned male at birth and has lived most of her life as a man. Martinez has been married to a woman for more than 40 years. She did not divulge her struggles with her assigned gender to her wife until she was in her late 20s. Her children did not find out until some years later, when they were in their late teens, due to Martinez's fear that they would reject her. She managed this by spending significant periods of time away from home to live as a woman. Martinez recalls coming out as a long process over years and talked movingly about the support she had received from her wife:

'So, we sat down, and she said, "let's go and have a meal together. You be yourself, Martinez and we'll meet somewhere away from home." So, we did. We told our children when they were all in their late teens, and their response was, "don't worry, it's alright, it's okay, it's absolutely fine, we understand, just come home to us". "How the bloody hell did you manage? Why didn't you tell us?" The children said, "what's the problem, why can't you be who you want to be?"'

Martinez told the researcher that she has decided not to transition fully, possibly reflecting her wife's stated needs to still see the person she married. Wanting to keep the relationship together is an important aspect of her later life experience. The couple had counselling and therapy and have met and supported other couples in similar situations. Martinez was adamant that partners/spouses need help to adjust, whether or not they want to continue the marriage. Crucially, this should not become marriage guidance, nor a way of overruling the wife's position, but what she termed "a safe environment" where partners can say what they feel, whatever they want or fear.

Martinez said: "It could be about diffusing anger, senses of betrayal, you know my wife said to me 'why didn't you tell me at the beginning?' I said it's because I thought it would go away." Martinez described how important sexual counselling was for her and her wife, particularly as her own identity was having an impact on her partner's sexual identity as they wanted to continue their intimate relationship. Martinez described the support she received from her peer group through a national charity and is aware from past experiences of the potential violence she could face in the public domain. However, she said she felt very privileged that her children responded well. They still call her dad, and because her grandchildren are so young, there has been no awkwardness whatsoever in her being able to affirm her gender identity and be herself around them.

What we can learn from these stories

Both of these stories illustrate the variety of different responses from family members that trans women experience when initially 'coming out' to members of their families. It reminds us that the process of 'coming out' is not a one-time event, and these experiences will have ongoing implications for relationships between all members of a family in the short and long term.

Martinez's comment about feeling privileged that her children responded so well is telling. She will be aware that not all trans women's experiences of coming out to their partner and children are as positive. Managing acrimony within family relationships is difficult; for the trans woman in the first story, following her 'coming out', her decision making about her own future was based on preserving relationships with her child and grandchildren at the expense of expressing her own sense of self. There are never right or wrong responses to these situations – but decisions will have intended and unintended consequences. The intended consequence for this trans woman was to have an ongoing relationship with members of her family. Acrimony in relationships can be toxic. However, the challenge to and potential loss of a relationship, particularly between a parent and child, can feel unbearable, hence decision making that affects a parent's willingness to express their gender diversity. This can be devastating for people who may have waited a long time to affirm their gender identity in later life. This may well have an impact or unintended consequences on an individual's own mental health in the longer term. Placing trans people in a position of choosing between expressing their authentic self and continuing a relationship with family members in the longer term as illustrated in both of these scenarios can be incredibly difficult and irresolvable where there might be no positive outcomes for the different parties.

Families and family structures are also forever changing. This can be for many reasons: people separate and end relationships, they create new partnerships, children are born into or join families, and as family members age, their needs change and relationships between family members change. Death also affects family relationships, and this may be something that trans individuals may be reflecting on as they get older if they have unresolved loss, longings, regrets and/or anger. The only thing that is guaranteed to be a constant force within families is change. In the case of Martinez and her family, we see communication and negotiations between family members – most notably Martinez and her wife. Honesty and compromise within these relationships has been core to them moving forward as a couple, and hopefully they will be able to support each other in later life. Martinez talked openly about the importance of her wife receiving support too. There are implications for her spouse in choosing to continue in a relationship with a partner whose gender identity has changed during the course of their relationship. These discussions have not been easy but have enabled Martinez to express herself openly and honestly in her relationships with her family members and has built trust and confidence in them.

The scenarios further allude to longer-term implications as both trans women get older and may need family support. The importance placed on relationships with children and grandchildren should not be underestimated but will vary over time and for each person. The consistent message for professionals is not to make assumptions but offer support and help to navigate these relationships as effectively as possible. For example, some older trans people may be asset rich and financially secure, but this does not translate to them having a vibrant social network to rely upon, and loneliness may still be a key concern (McNeil et al, 2012). This is illustrated positively for Martinez and her wife, whereas this was less effective in the first scenario.

Conclusion

Later life brings challenges in which families are often relied upon or assumed to be able to be relied upon to help with any care needs. This is often the cornerstone of government social policy. Many studies have examined the effects of social support from children on older adults' subjective wellbeing (Cheng et al, 2013; Bangerteret et al, 2015) and have shown that older parents and their children receiving and providing support enhances subjective wellbeing, particularly if this is founded on reciprocity (Toyoshima and Nakahara, 2021). In the general population, objective measures of social isolation, subjective feelings of loneliness and living alone are all known to be associated with increased mortality and worse health outcomes (Holt-Lunstad et al, 2015). The development of caring relationships, both within families and within trans communities, is therefore an important factor in resilience and wellbeing in later life (McFadden et al, 2013). However, given the evidence on higher levels of family estrangement in trans populations, this is likely to lead to less access to support networks and a reduction in protective or mitigating factors to support both physical and mental health wellbeing (Fredriksen-Goldsen et al, 2014).

Understanding trans people's social support networks in later life is an important aspect of good assessments and should inform interventions that can promote and enhance good health and help to mitigate the impact of minority stress. A study of trans and gender non-binary (TGNB) older people's experiences during the COVID-19 lockdown in the UK and Australia (Toze et al, 2023b) identified that the main source of social support during such a time of uncertainty and crisis was provided by friends, followed by family and then LGBT+/trans-specific support groups only. However, 14 per cent of participants said they had no support networks. The majority of trans and gender non-conforming (TGNC) UK survey participants in this study reported living alone, but many discussed diverse and active social support networks. While friends tended to be most frequently highlighted as sources of support, there were also references to the importance of intimate partners, adult children, other family members and neighbours. Many TGNC participants in this study also discussed participation in a range of social and community activities, including LGBT/trans-specific organisations as well as a range of other faith, community and hobby activities (Toze et al, 2023b).

We have seen from a review of the empirical literature that there is limited evidence on trans ageing trajectories in relation to parenting and family life. Trans parents face complexities when exploring and negotiating their gender identities within the context of their existing family relationships and personal commitments. The two stories outlined earlier illustrate the diversity of experiences within these trajectories and some of the issues that mediate or cumulate future access to support in later life (Pearce, 2018; Toze, 2019). We know that the compounded effects of minority stress are closely connected with outcomes for older trans people (Testa et al, 2012; Westwood et al, 2020), but trans lives and experiences of family care in relation to parenting have been marginalised from this analytical framework. Exploring the parenting and caring experiences of trans people from a life course perspective that accounts for ageing could enable a richer understanding of the construction and experiences of caring, parenting and gender, essential to person-centred support (Hines, 2006; 2007).

In these scenarios, formal channels of support through health and social care professionals, such as counsellors or psychologists experienced in working with families, are important. However, the serious dearth of specialist knowledge and skills needs to be addressed in professional education, in the commissioning of mainstream services and not least investment in peer-informed and led support systems (Hafford-Letchfield et al, 2020). Further longitudinal research on trans people and their families will help to understand the needs of trans parents, co-parents and their children over the life span to take account of ageing and other milestones in later life (Charter et al, 2023). Other family members such as siblings have also been observed to be an important source of support (Riggs, 2016), and these generational differences may also be important when discussing the relationship between trans individuals and their families (Borges et al, 2022). Professionals should deconstruct and challenge normative assumptions about how families form, support each other and what that support might look like. A narrative approach (Bower et al, 2021) that helps to articulate themes of generativity and resilience and what we can learn from experiences, or the application of techniques to map support networks, can help to emphasise autonomy and build a supportive environment for the older trans person and their whole 'family' system, including families of choice (de Brito Silver et al, 2023).

Further, the idea of family, particularly more traditional views on the nuclear family, is one that needs to be deconstructed to take account of shifting gender identities and recognise that family acceptance is different from family support (Borges et al, 2022). Trans older people may for example need support beyond acceptance to be able to navigate other challenges in their lives such as unemployment and changes in health and care needs. It can be challenging for a trans older person to exercise choices about care when their financial resources are limited and the impact of earlier discrimination in employment and family conflict can be cumulative in relation to limited options and resources. Society often promotes positive images of having a supportive family in later life, but there are minoritised communities within trans populations who have a long trajectory of family abandonment and rejection complicated by other identities such as disability, ethnicity and sexual identity (Silva et al, 2023). Increasing numbers of more genderfluid and non-binary older people will likely require more active engagement with care services and different family relationships.

Despite significant shifts in legislative, political, cultural and social contexts, which have improved our understanding of diverse gender identities and family life, specific issues for older trans people remain underexplored within healthcare, social work and social care. As we saw in the scenarios in this chapter, some trans individuals' transition may be ongoing and something they are continually negotiating. Trans older people's parenting experiences have been marginalised within mainstream professional practice, and action is required to address these inequalities to challenge social policy when providing care and social support. We conclude with some brief points for practice.

Summary learning points

- Focus on early intervention and education to support relationships with family members such as children, grandchildren and families of choice when a parent is affirming their gender identity, regardless of their age.
- For trans older people living alone with experiences of family estrangement, consider what interventions might be developed to help them build links with others, for example via third sector or community organisations who have a good understanding of their needs.
- Professionals and providers should pay more attention to gaining the knowledge and skills needed to support a trans older individual with their parenting, grandparenting and family relationships where the person wants or asks for this. Focus on human rights and tailor work to the specific individual. Affirming the diversity of family life requires that professionals take active responsibility and be more accountable in educating themselves and others on these rights.
- Reach out to the trans community to include them in accessing and improving services for families who may be adapting to change or in dispute and in turn be active with trans organisations to ensure that family services are inclusive, responsive and age sensitive to their needs.

References

Bangerter, L.R., Kim, K., Zarit, S.H., Birditt, K.S. and Fingerman, K.L. (2015) 'Perceptions of giving support and depressive symptoms in late life', *The Gerontologist*, 55(5): 770–9.

Barnes, J., Breckon, M.R., Houle, K., Morgan, R., Paquette, M. and Taylor, C. (2006) 'Nowhere near enough: a needs assessment of health and safety services for transgender and two spirit people in Manitoba and Northwestern Ontario', Crime Prevention Branch Public Safety and Emergency Preparedness Canada, Available from: https://ninecircles.ca/wp-content/uploads/2017/04/Trans-Needs-Assessment-Full-Report.pdf

Bouman, W.P., Claes, L., Marshall, E., Pinner, G.T, Longworth, J., Maddox, V. et al (2016) 'Socio-demographic variables, clinical features, and the role of preassessment cross-sex hormones in older trans people', *Journal of Sexual Medicine*, 13(4): 711–19.

Bower, K.L, Lewis, D.C, Bermúdez, J.M. and Singh, A.A. (2021) 'Narratives of generativity and resilience among LGBT older adults: leaving positive legacies despite social stigma and collective trauma', *Journal of Homosexuality*, 68(2): 230–51.

Carone, N., Rothblum, E.D., Bos, H.M.W., Gartrell, N.K. and Herman, J.L. (2021) 'Demographics and health outcomes in a U.S. probability sample of transgender parents', *Journal of Family Psychology*, 35(1): 57–68.

Charter, R., Ussher, J.M., Perz, J. and Robinson, K.H. (2023) 'Transgender parents: negotiating "coming out" and gender affirmation with children and co-parents', *Journal of Homosexuality*, 70(7): 1287–309.

Cheng, Y.P., Birditt, K.S., Zarit, S.H. and Fingerman, K.L. (2013) 'Young adults' provision of support to middle-aged parents', *The Journals of Gerontology: Series B; Psychological Sciences and Social Sciences*, 70(3): 407–16.

Cocker, C. (2022) 'Lesbian parenting: rebellious or conformist', in C. Cocker and T. Hafford-Letchfield (eds) *Rethinking Feminist Theories for Social Work Practice*, Cham: Palgrave Macmillan, pp 271–86.

Cosby, R. and Berry-Edwards, J. (2022) 'Economic security and family well-being', in *Encyclopaedia of Social Work*, Oxford: Oxford University Press, Available from: https://oxfordre.com/socialwork/

Danilo Borges, P., Pastor-Valero, M. and Machin, R. (2022) '"This family rejection harmed my health as well": intersections between the meanings of family and health for trans people and family members in a trans healthcare service in Brazil', *Global Public Health*, 17(7): 1330–42.

De Brito Silva, B., Vaitses Fontanari, A.M., Seibel, B.L., Chinazzo, Í.R., Luxion, K., Rodrigues Lobato, M.I. et al (2023) 'Transgender parenthood, participation in children's lives, and association with discrimination experiences: an exploratory study', *Family Relations*, 72(1): 122–39.

Diener, E. and Seligman, M.E.P. (2002) 'Very happy people', *Psychological Science*, 13(1): 81–4.

Donovan, C., Heaphy, B. and Weeks, J. (2001) *Same Sex Intimacies: Families of Choice and Other Life Experiments*, London: Routledge.

Fredriksen-Goldsen, K.I., Simoni, J.M., Kim, H.-J., Lehavot, K., Walters, K.L., Yang, J. et al (2014) 'The health equity promotion model: reconceptualization of lesbian, gay, bisexual, and transgender (LGBT) health disparities', *The American Journal of Orthopsychiatry*, 84(6): 653–63.

Freedman, D., Tasker, F. and di Ceglie, D. (2002) 'Children and adolescents with transsexual parents referred to a specialist gender identity development service: a brief report of key developmental features', *Clinical Child Psychology and Psychiatry*, 7(3): 423–32.

Government Equalities Office (2018) 'National LGBT survey: research report', Available from: https://assets.publishing.service.gov.uk/government/uploads/system/uploads/attachment_data/file/722314/GEO-LGBT-Survey-Report.pdf

Grant, J.M., Mottet, L., Tanis, J.E., Harrison, J., Herman, J. and Keisling, M. (2011) 'Injustice at every turn: a report of the National Transgender Discrimination Survey', Washington, DC: National Center for Transgender Equality and National Gay and Lesbian Task Force.

Hafford-Letchfield, T., Cocker, C., Rutter, D., Manning, R. and McCormack, K. (2021) 'Doing the right thing and getting it right: professional perspectives in social work on supporting parents from gender diverse communities', *International Journal of Transgender Health*, 22(1–2): 154–66.

Hafford-Letchfield, T., Cocker, C., Rutter, D., Tinarwo, M., McCormack, K. and Manning, R. (2019) 'What do we know about transgender parenting? Findings from a systematic review', *Health and Social Care in the Community*, 27(5): 1111–25.

Haines, B.A., Ajayi, A.A. and Boyd, H. (2014) 'Making trans parents visible: intersectionality of trans and parenting identities', *Feminism & Psychology*, 24(2): 238–47.

Health Foundation (2021) 'Our ageing population: how ageing affects health and social care in England', London: Health Foundation.

Herman, J.L. (2014) 'Gendered restrooms and minority stress: the public regulation of gender and its impact on transgender people's lives', UCLA School of Law: Williams Institute, pp 65–80.

Hines, S. (2006) 'Intimate transitions: transgender practices of partnering and parenting', *Sociology: The Journal of the British Sociological Association*, 40(2): 353–71.

Hines, S. (2007) 'Transgendering care: practices of care within transgender communities', *Critical Social Policy*, 27(4): 462–86.

Holt-Lunstad, J., Smith, T.B, Baker, M., Harris, T. and Stephenson D. (2015) 'Loneliness and social isolation as risk factors for mortality: a meta-analytic review', *Perspectives in Psychological Science*, 10(2): 227–37.

McFadden, S.H., Frankowski, S., Flick, H. and Witten, T.M. (2013) 'Resilience and multiple stigmatized identities: lessons from transgender persons' reflections on aging', in J.D. Sinnott (ed) *Positive Psychology: Advances in Understanding Adult Motivation*, New York: Springer, pp 247–67, Available from: https://doi.org/10.1007/978-1-4614-7282-7_16

McNeil, J., Bailey, L., Ellis, S., Morton, J. and Regan, M. (2012) 'Trans mental health study, 2012', Scottish Transgender Alliance, Sheffield Hallam University, Available from: https://www.scottishtrans.org/wp-content/uploads/2013/03/trans_mh_study.pdf

Pyne, J., Bauer, G. and Bradley, K. (2015) 'Transphobia and other stressors impacting trans parents', *Journal of GLBT Family Studies*, 11(2): 107–26.

Riggs, D.W., Power, J. and von Doussa, H. (2016) 'Parenting and Australian trans and gender diverse people: an exploratory survey', *International Journal of Transgenderism*, 17(2): 59–65.

Stotzer, R.L., Herman, J.L. and Hasenbush, A. (2014) 'Transgender parenting: a review of existing research', Los Angeles: Williams Institute.

Testa, R.J., Sciacca, L.M., Wang, F., Hendricks, M.L., Goldblum, P., Bradford, J. et al (2012) 'Effects of violence on transgender people', *Professional Psychology: Research and Practice*, 43(5): 452–9.

Toyoshima, A. and Nakahara, J. (2021) 'The effects of familial social support relationships on identity meaning in older adults: a longitudinal investigation', *Frontiers in Psychology*, 12: e50051, Available from: https://doi.org/10.3389/fpsyg.2021.650051

Toze, M. (2019) 'Developing a critical trans gerontology', *British Journal of Sociology*, 70(4): 1490–509. DOI: 10.1111/1468-4446.12491.

Toze, M., Gates, T.G., Hughes, M., Dune, T., Westwood, S., Hafford-Letchfield, T. et al (2023a) 'Social support in older transgender and gender diverse communities in the United Kingdom and Australia: a comparative study during COVID-19', *Journal of Gerontological Social Work*, 66(3): 381–99.

Toze, M., Westwood, S. and Hafford-Letchfield, T. (2023b) 'Social support and unmet needs among older trans and gender non-conforming people during the COVID-19 "lockdown" in the UK', *International Journal of Transgender Health*, 24(3): 305–19. DOI: 10.1080/26895269.2021.1977210.

Veldorale-Griffin, A. (2014) 'Transgender parents and their adult children's experiences of disclosure and transition', *Journal of GLBT Family Studies*, 10(5): 475–501.

Veldorale-Griffin, A. and Darling, C.A. (2016) 'Adaptation to parental gender transition: stress and resilience among transgender parents', *Archives of Sexual Behavior*, 45: 607–17, Available from: https://doi.org/10.1007/s10508-015-0657-3

Von Doussa, H., Power, J. and Riggs, D. (2015) 'Imagining parenthood: the possibilities and experiences of parenthood among transgender people', *Culture Health & Sexuality*, 17(9): 1119–31.

Westwood, S., Willis, P., Fish, J., Hafford-Letchfield, T., Semelyan, J., King, A. et al (2020) 'Older LGBT+ health inequalities in the UK: setting a research agenda', *Journal of Epidemiological Community Health*, 74(5): 408–11.

White, T. and Ettner, R. (2004) 'Disclosure, risks, and protective factors for children whose parents are undergoing a gender transition', *Journal of Gay & Lesbian Psychotherapy*, 8(1–2): 129–45.

5

"What happened to my body over the past decade?" Trans masculine ageing and embodiment in a cisgenderist and ageist society

Alexandre Baril

Introduction: subjective affects and experiences of embodiment in cisgenderist and ageist contexts

"Hey girls!" said one of my colleagues, a few years ago, as he walked past my office while I was working with a female colleague.[1] This greeting would have gone unnoticed if I was a woman. But as a binary trans man who transitioned 15 years ago, who has not been misgendered for over a decade by people who didn't know me before my transition, and who is always correctly gendered in my interactions with strangers based on my masculine appearance and gender expression, this interpellation left me speechless and unable to defend myself against this violent act of misgendering. "Hey girls! ..." "Hey girls! ..." To this day, I am still haunted by those two simple words, echoing in my head and heart, pounding, always louder, to the point of not hearing my own thoughts, to the point of sometimes not feeling the euphoria that my transition brought into my life, numbed by the weight of those words that shattered my masculinity.

It must be said that this incident was part of a series of several misgendering instances that happened suddenly, around four years ago, in my department of social work, a small department composed of 15 faculty members and a few administrative staff. At the time, I had been employed there for over a year. While I cannot know for sure what propelled those unexpected occurrences of misgendering by approximately a third of the department, I can say that this arrived after some fraught discussions on equity, diversity and inclusion issues during which I expressed disagreement with colleagues. It must be said that these colleagues also know that I am a trans, bisexual and disabled/Mad[2] man, since I was hired as a specialist of queer/trans and disability/Mad studies, and I have always been transparent about my identities. Contrary to the strangers I encounter in my public interactions – be it at the grocery store, mall or restaurant – who read me as a cisgender man based on what Julia Serano (2007, p 164) calls 'cissexual assumption', presuming that I was assigned male at birth and granting me cissexual privilege – my colleagues knew that I was trans and, based on that fact, took away those cis privileges from me. In other words, I only have 'conditional cissexual privilege' (Serano, 2007, p 169), effective and granted precisely when people don't know that I am trans. Otherwise, those cis privileges can be denied, and forms of misgendering and delegitimisation of gender identity can occur based on people's 'cissexual gender entitlement' (Serano, 2007, p 165). In that sense, "Hey girls!" is the epitome of this denial of my masculine gender identity. Like the other misgendering incidents that happened for over a year at the office, right before the COVID-19 pandemic hit, it illustrates the cisgenderist and cisnormative[3] contexts within which trans and gender diverse people are confined. To adapt the well-known trope 'trapped in the wrong body', trans and gender diverse people are trapped in the wrong societies that deny their self-determination and self-identification.

This "Hey girls!" incident crystallised the starting point of a personal quest for what we call 'top surgery' (mastectomy) in trans communities. While I transitioned socially, legally and medically starting in 2008, and have completed several surgeries since then, I have never had top surgery. I am one of the rare transmasculine people who didn't need a mastectomy to give my chest an appearance coded as masculine. When I started my transition, I barely had breasts, and the combination of testosterone hormonal therapy and bodybuilding provided me with masculine pectorals, to the point of going bare chested at the pool or the beach without intrusive gazes, and even receiving several compliments throughout the years about my muscular upper body and chest. But now being a middle-aged man in my mid-40s, my body has slowly started to change. Despite not having gained substantial weight, my fat distribution and fat deposits have changed slightly with age, as well as my skin elasticity, among other corporeal changes. What seemed to me to be the perfect pectorals ten years ago have now started looking like tiny 'man boobs', a reality I also see occurring for many middle-aged and older cisgender/cis men I know personally or see in the public sphere (a condition called gynecomastia that affects about between 32 per cent and 65 per cent of all cis men and about half of cis men above 50 years old; see Holzmer et al, 2020). While there is no doubt that many of those middle-aged and older cis men, in an ageist society that valorises youth and muscular, lean and fit bodies have a hard time accepting their changing bodies, as evidenced by the staggering number of gynecomastia (or breast reduction) surgeries performed on cis men (Holzmer et al, 2020), the significance of this transformation of my body is noteworthy from a trans perspective. Although many cis men might feel their masculinity is called into question when they fail to meet ageist, heterosexist or ableist norms (Siverskog, 2015; Baril and Silverman, 2019), such questioning of masculinity takes a particular toll on trans men in cisgenderist and cisnormative contexts that deny their masculine identity (Toze, 2021). It is in this cisgenderist and ageist context, and following the "Hey girls!" interpellation, that I started doubting the fragile sense of masculinity I had built over the years. At the time, I started to wonder if my hormones had stopped working, or if the corporeal changes brought by age were giving my body a different look and gendered expression. Despite being reassured that this was not the case by people in my life, and even by surgeons in private clinics (with financial incentive to encourage surgeries) who told me that my chest looked better than most cis men and they would not consider doing the surgery if they were me, I kept obsessing over my chest, to the point of now being on a waiting list for a surgery in a clinic offering free surgeries in my province (Quebec). The "Hey girls!" moment translates how social violence can become intertwined with the corporeal and subjective processes of ageing, literally carving itself into the body and the skin and scarring the mind, heart and flesh.

Founded on an autoethnographic methodology (Ellis et al, 2011), and building on and extending scholarship in critical trans gerontology (Toze, 2019) and intersectionality put forth by Black feminists, who pointed out how various identities and their related oppressions, such as sexism and racism, are interlocked (Crenshaw, 1989; Hill Collins, 2000), this chapter focuses on my own navigation of ageing as a trans man in order to offer broader reflections regarding middle-aged trans men to help healthcare professionals better support trans middle-aged and older people. These reflections are important for initiating dialogues between scholars from various disciplines, such as critical gerontology, masculinity studies and trans studies, as well as among practitioners, who must engage in conversation to address inequality in ageing. The remainder of this chapter is divided into three parts. The first points to some limitations in the literature on trans ageing. The second, based on an autoethnographic account anchored in my experience as a trans middle-aged man, provides personal narratives that can help healthcare professionals better comprehend the complex intersections of transness and ageing and cisgenderism and ageism. The third insists on the importance, for academics and practitioners, of endorsing an intersectional approach to better serve marginalised populations living at the intersection of multiple oppressions.

Missing conversations in trans gerontological literature

As a rapidly evolving field, trans gerontology has focused on the challenges, barriers and discriminations faced by trans older adults, particularly in relation to healthcare and social services, as well as in various institutional settings (Hébert et al, 2013; Cook-Daniels, 2015; Porter et al, 2016; Hardacker et al, 2019; Nowakowski et al, 2021). This literature describes the micro-aggressions (for example misgendering) and structural cisgenderist violence encountered by trans older adults and their impacts on physical and mental health (Witten, 2003; Fredriksen-Goldsen et al, 2014; Ansara, 2015; Cook-Daniels, 2015; Porter et al, 2016; Bailey et al, 2019; Willis et al, 2021). This body of scholarship also discusses several social determinants of health that impact ageing processes for trans people living at the intersection of various marginalised identities (Witten, 2003; Cook-Daniels, 2015; Pang et al, 2019). Many studies address the isolation and lack of support for older trans people (Siverskog, 2014; Cook-Daniels, 2015; Latham and Barrett, 2015; Pang et al, 2019), including their marginalisation within larger LGBTQ communities and organisations (Fabbre and Siverskog, 2020). Others focus on trans people's fears and concerns about ageing, including those pertaining to dementia (Latham and Barrett, 2015; Baril and Silverman, 2019; Bishop and Westwood, 2019; Pearce, 2019; Silverman and Baril, 2021, 2023) and end-of-life planning (Bailey, 2012; Witten and Eyler, 2012; Pang et al, 2019). Almost all scholarship insists on the need for more knowledge on the topic, particularly among healthcare professionals (Bailey, 2012; Siverskog, 2014; Porter et al, 2016; Toze, 2019; Nowakowski et al, 2021; Benbow et al, 2022), and some provide concrete recommendations for healthcare professionals to better serve trans older adults (Hébert et al, 2013; Ansara, 2015; Porter et al, 2016; Nowakowski et al, 2021).

Limitations of the current literature

In a seminal article on 'critical trans gerontology', Michael Toze (2019) highlights the strengths of this literature as well as its limitations. For example, Toze (2019, p 1499) shows that 'there is relatively little data on trans people's experiences of ageing. We know little about how trans people experience age-related bodily change, ageism, or key moments in later stages of the lifecourse.' Toze also stresses that despite its reference to concepts such as intersectionality, this literature does 'not necessarily address in theoretical depth how such concepts can be applied to trans experiences' (p 1491). I concur with Toze's observations, and the literature reviewed here, and for previous texts (Baril and Silverman, 2019; Silverman and Baril, 2021), allows me to point to three gaps in this scholarship: (1) the under-theorisation of the experiences of middle-aged trans people; (2) the lack of focus on specific genders, such as masculine or feminine trans people; (3) the lack of tools and concrete examples to better understand trans ageing trajectories from an intersectional perspective. I address each of these gaps in turn.

First, while trans gerontology is characterised by its inclusion of 'younger' ageing people in research – with most research projects including adults of 50 years of age or older (for example: Fabbre, 2014; Bailey et al, 2019; Fabbre and Gaveras, 2020; Willis et al, 2021) – studies often focus on the realities of those who have retired, who live in care homes, who experience multiple health issues, who live with dementia and so forth. Despite some exceptions (Witten, 2003; Witten and Eyler, 2012; Nowakowski et al, 2021; Toze, 2021; Willis et al, 2021), very few studies discuss issues faced by middle-aged people. However, while some trans middle-aged people might face similar hurdles to older ones, they also have distinctive experiences of ageing that justify the need for more research on the specific realities of middle-aged trans adults. Second, surprisingly few studies in trans gerontology address the specific realities of each gender: transfeminine, transmasculine and gender diverse people's realities are often discussed indistinguishably (Toze, 2021). Consequently, the specific experiences of transmasculine people remain under-theorised (Toze, 2021). Third, despite the stated commitment to intersectionality, concrete intersectional analyses of the lived experiences of trans older adults remain scarce. With a few exceptions (Siverskog, 2014, 2015; Baril and Silverman, 2019; Pearce, 2019; Toze, 2019, 2021; Silverman and Baril, 2021, 2023), scholarship often reiterates that various components of identity and oppression are interlocked yet don't offer concrete illustrations of how transness and ageing, and cisgenderism and ageism, intersect.

An intersectional approach to the current literature

Despite its limitations, the literature available at the time of writing this chapter points to some interesting intersectional angles on which can be built a more comprehensive portrait of the interlocking identity components of trans and ageing and their related oppressions. A first angle examines how age(ing) impacts transness, through its implications on gender performance (Siverskog, 2014, 2015). While not wanting to associate ageing with decline, many older people experience physiological changes that might impact their gendered performance or alter the way people perceive their gender in our ageist and sexist/cisgenderist society, such as changes in fat distribution and body hair colour and texture. In my case, the least invasive top surgery, for which I am currently a good candidate, will not be available to me indefinitely: I have a temporal window of about five years, a period after which I will most likely, due to ageing, have lost too much skin elasticity and be forced to have a more invasive procedure. A second angle scrutinises the impacts of transness on age(ing). Trans people often experience non-normative ways of aging and a non-linear life course (Fabbre, 2014; Siverskog, 2015; Pearce, 2019; Toze, 2021). Those who undergo medical treatments, including hormone therapy, experience a second puberty (Bailey, 2012; Ansara, 2015; Siverskog, 2015; Pearce, 2019; Toze, 2021; Willis et al, 2021). People transitioning at an older age might also have a sense of a 'new beginning' (Pang et al, 2019, p 50) and a new relationship to temporality (Willis et al, 2021).

Additionally, lifelong experiences of cisgenderism, micro-aggressions and minority stress can take a toll on trans older adults and provoke premature ageing (Witten, 2003; Hébert, Enriquez and Chamberland, 2013). A third angle puts the emphasis on how ageist structures interact with, and amplify, cisgenderism. Presumptions about older people, which often associate old age with physical and cognitive decline, tend to reinforce cisgenderism and medical gatekeeping regarding transitions (Siverskog, 2014, 2015; Baril and Silverman, 2019). For example, excuses related to presumed precarious health in later life (for example disability, chronic illness) are used to deny trans older people surgeries or hormones (Hébert et al, 2013; Willis et al, 2021; Silverman and Baril, 2023). A fourth angle conceptualises the impacts of cisgenderism on ageism. Indeed, the gatekeeping and paternalism faced by trans people in healthcare can, in return, reinforce the paternalism directed at older people. The multidirectional links between transness and ageing and cisgenderism and ageism take different forms. In the remainder of this chapter, I offer personal narratives addressing my experience of trans ageing to better understand those multidirectional links.

"What happened to my body over the past decade?": an autoethnographic account of trans masculine ageing

Autoethnography specialists Carolyn Ellis and colleagues identify various forms of autoethnography, anchored in Indigenous, narrative, reflexive and community ethnographies or personal narratives, as methodological tools allowing researchers to mobilise subjective experience to exemplify broader social contexts, experiences, structures and norms. They describe how autoethnographies that rest upon personal narratives allow the readers to learn from the autoethnographer's situated perspective and conceptualise their own experiences in the light of those proposed by the author. The generalisability of autoethnographies must be understood from a different lens than a positivist/postpositivist epistemology:

> In autoethnography, the focus of generalizability moves from respondents to readers, and is always being tested by readers as they determine if a story speaks to them about their experience or about the lives of others they know; it is determined by whether the (specific) autoethnographer is able to illuminate (general) unfamiliar cultural processes. (Ellis et al, 2011: np)

While the reflections proposed here are not representative of the multiplicity of trans and gender diverse people's realities and are applicable only to a subset of trans people – those who identify as binary transmasculine and go through a medical transition – I believe that sharing my personal narrative can illuminate more broadly the complex relationships between transness and ageing and cisgenderism and ageism.

In the spirit of Toze's (2019, p 1500) invitation to value life stories and personal narratives to better grasp 'subjective notions of ageing', I return here to two components of my identity (transness and ageing) and their related oppressions. The fact that I am White, educated and part of the upper class as a tenured professor, along with the fact that I am disabled/Mad, are not taken into consideration. This doesn't mean that those other components don't play a significant role in my trans ageing process, quite the contrary. Yet for the purpose of this demonstration, I 'strategically selected' transness and ageing as 'anchor points' of my intersectional analysis (Toze, 2019, p 1500), since the subjective experiences of trans ageing remain under-documented, particularly for trans men (Toze, 2019, 2021).

Middle age is a period of significant bodily change for cis and trans people, and I observe this vividly in my case. First, as a disabled person who has been living with chronic pain for over 15 years and is used to managing the fatigue that comes with pain, I have noticed that my energy level is not at the same as it used to be. I now tire more easily, and I cannot accomplish as many things in a day as I used to when I was younger. This has consequences on some practices, including physical activities and workouts. Needless to say, activities such as workouts represent gender(ed) technologies that are part of practices that shape the gendered self. The results are quantifiable: I had to reduce the number of exercises I do and the weight I am capable of lifting to avoid injuries or pain. These changes to my workout routine have impacted my body shape, and while my body is still coded as masculine by dominant standards, the 'quest for size' often shared by cis and trans men in sexist and heterosexist society is impacted by ageing.

A second important change that occurs over time, for many people including myself, is the accumulation of fat deposits in some parts of the body. As fat studies scholars remind us, fat is highly gendered: not only does the interpretation of fatness vary according to gender norms but fatness and slenderness contribute to the construction of gendered bodies. Fat and trans scholar Francis Ray White (2014, p 90) writes that 'for transmasculine people, fatness often appears as threatening because it is perceived as feminizing. Ridding the body of feminine curves and fleshiness is constructed as an important aspect of attaining a more masculine embodiment.' As disability scholars have shown that disability undoes gender and desexualises disabled people in our ableist and sexist societies (Baril and Silverman, 2019; Silverman and Baril, 2021), a similar phenomenon is at play when it comes to size status in fatphobic contexts: fatness contributes to degendering and desexualising cis and trans people. But, as White reminds us, this is particularly significant for fat trans people in a society that delegitimises their gender identification. Let's recall, as mentioned earlier, that about half of cis men over 50 years old experience enlarged breasts due to an increase of glandular tissue or fat tissue (Holzmer et al, 2020). In my case, the combination of my glandular breast tissue with an increase of fat deposits in this area has modified the appearance of my pectorals. That change is intertwined with another change that comes with ageing: skin texture and the loss of skin elasticity over time (wrinkles and sagginess). All these changes due to ageing have slowly but surely impacted the look of my chest. While these changes are likely imperceptible to most, being a trans man in a cisgenderist society that invalidates trans masculinity deeply impacts the way I experience my ageing body and chest.

Following the autoethnographic reflections that White (2014) offers on the complex intersections of transness and fatness to conceptualise his desire for a flat chest as a fat trans person, I apply some of those considerations to transness and ageing. White (2014, p 92) argues that both trans and fat studies have theorised the importance of 'being at home' in one's body, yet from very different perspectives. In trans studies, being at home means accepting the potential transformations of your body (for example, through hormone therapy, surgery, exercise or gender expression), but, in fat studies, it means maintaining your body as it is while transforming your perceptions of your body and fighting fatphobic societies. White (2014, p 93) asks the following question: 'what do these conflicting discourses [of fat and trans studies on embodiment] offer someone who is both fat and trans in terms of their hope of feeling "at home" in their body?' White (2014, p 96) concludes that

> [t]he 'flat chest' so desired by FTMs [Female-to-Male] and other transmasculine people, myself included, is as much a slender bodily ideal as it is a non-feminine one. A queer perspective might problematize how moves to acquire a flat chest may work to reproduce the norms that feminize fat cisgendered males and make their 'moobs' (man-boobs) an object of ridicule, as well as the targets of gender-policing weight-loss regimes.

Like White, I have found myself trapped, not in the wrong body, but at the intersection of not only transness and ageing, and cisgenderism and ageism, but also of anti-ageist and trans-affirmative discourses on embodiment. In a similar fashion to fat studies, critical gerontology discourses, through the historical dominance of a script of accepting and celebrating the ageing body, has insisted on changing oneself and society's perception of the body instead of promoting individual corporeal changes to maintain a young body and appearance. This insistence on keeping the body as it is and transforming (internalised) societal norms about older bodies has, in some ways, cast critical gerontology's ambitions regarding embodiment as different from trans studies' understanding of embodiment as malleable. While trans studies and movements certainly fight for transforming cisgenderist and cisnormative societies to broaden our imagination about gender identities and expressions, they have also advocated for the importance of self-determination and the possibility of bodily transformation. If we return to White's question in this context, we could ask: what do the conflicting discourses on embodiment of critical gerontology and trans studies offer someone who is both older and trans, in terms of their hope of feeling at home in their body? In my case, it translates into my desire, as a scholar in critical gerontology, to accept and celebrate my ageing body (including its sagginess and changes in fat distribution in my chest), as well as my desire, as a trans activist and scholar, to celebrate the malleability of the body and the empowerment that can come through modifying bodily features. I am aware that the desire for older transmasculine people to have a flat and firm chest rests upon both an ageist bodily ideal and a non-feminine one. And while these two identities and realities, being trans and older, are not contradictory, the fact that transness and ageing have been (under-)conceptualised over the past decades has forced trans older people to think about their identities and oppressions in silo, rather than as intertwined.

Furthermore, the subjective experience of embodiment can never be dissociated from its sociopolitical aspects. Healthcare professionals should therefore pay close attention, in their interactions with trans middle-aged and older adults, to how ageing processes impact gender identity and expression (and vice-versa) and how complex forces are at play through normative forms of embodiment based on age and gender. As previously mentioned, my recent desire for a top surgery goes beyond the impacts that the ageing process has had on my body and gender identity. Indeed, the desire for surgery first occurred in the context of cisgenderist violence I experienced professionally. To add to this complexity, the misgendering I experienced cannot be separated from my linguistic context. As the French language (my first language and the language used in my department) is more gendered than English, opportunities to misgender go far beyond the usage of the wrong pronouns or interpellations such as "Hey girls!" Adjectives and nouns in French are most often gendered. To give only one example, a student in French needs to be designated as masculine (*étudiant*) or feminine (*étudiante*), and no noun exists to designate a non-gendered student. This leaves room for a lot of misgendering occasions, since the nouns and adjectives used in every sentence are coded as masculine or feminine. In sum, it is impossible to separate linguistic cisgenderist micro-aggressions from my subjective experience of embodiment.

The impacts of COVID-19 on trans wellbeing and body image

A further layer of complexity is the broader social context in which my desire for a top surgery is anchored. Indeed, the episodes of misgendering

I explained earlier occurred just before the COVID-19 pandemic began in 2020. When the pandemic hit, my university switched to online teaching and activities. On the one hand, working remotely provided me with a measure of protection from my toxic workplace environment by reducing my interaction with colleagues. On the other hand, online working amplified my desire for surgery by altering my perspective of my body as a result of looking at myself through videoconferencing technologies. While it is not my intention here to discuss the literature documenting the impacts of COVID-19 and the increased usage of technologies on people's physical and mental health and body image, it is noteworthy to mention that for many of us, the usage of those technologies transformed the way we relate to ourselves and to our bodies. For example, when I teach in person, I am usually standing up and don't see my own body or image. However, when teaching, supervising or meeting on Zoom, I have a different point of view on my body. First, I am sitting down, and this position gives the upper body a different look, be it through posture or the way creases of clothing appear on the chest. Second, while videoconferencing, you look at others *as well as at yourself*, a phenomenon that can call attention to bodily details that might otherwise have gone unnoticed. I therefore spent the past three years on Zoom looking at the appearance of my chest. It is interesting to note that this continuous virtual gaze occurred right after the events that contributed to the fragilisation of my sense of masculinity. This also happens in a pandemic context where I have been systematically wearing a mask for the past three years when I go out, a practice that, as some recent research has shown (Dubois et al, 2022), generates anxiety and concerns among transmasculine people for whom wearing a mask increases misgendering due to the invisibility of facial hair under the mask. In sum, my desire for a top surgery is enmeshed in a complex web of factors: while some are more 'factual', such as fat deposits or saggy skin due to ageing, these can never be dissociated from the social contexts, structures and norms that construct these subjectivities.

Conclusion: the value of an intersectional approach to trans ageing

By offering this contextualised and personal account of the socio-subjective components intertwined in my desire for a top surgery, this chapter proposes tools to begin remedying the three limitations previously identified in trans gerontology literature. Those limitations leave academics, activists, trans (and) older people, as well as healthcare professionals, poorly equipped to understand the lived experience of trans and gender diverse older people from an intersectional perspective. An intersectional lens would help practitioners better intervene with trans and gender diverse people of all ages or older people of all genders that live at the intersection of other oppressions.

Non-intersectional ways of conceptualising and dealing with trans older adults can take various forms. For example, if we go back to my experience, the gender identity clinic offering me a free top surgery requires a letter from a therapist confirming a diagnosis of gender dysphoria. A few months after submitting the required documents, the clinic contacted me to indicate that my therapist's letter was invalid, since it stated that I *seem* to present gender dysphoria instead of *have* gender dysphoria. While expressing my dissatisfaction with their excessive gatekeeping process that required me to ask my therapist for a new letter with one word changed, I complied with the request. The 'funny' thing is that I don't currently have gender dysphoria and never had dysphoria in relation to my chest. First, my gender identity and body have been masculine for the past 15 years. Second, my chest has been a source of both pleasure in my sexuality and pride, either when I 'pass' as a cis person and receive compliments on my upper body, or when I receive comments from transmasculine people impressed with my scarless chest. However, the healthcare professionals, from a non-intersectional perspective, often insist on the importance of a diagnosis of gender dysphoria (Willis et al, 2021), a view that doesn't consider other factors such as ageing (or cisgenderism and ageism), among many others, that might play a greater role than gender dysphoria in my decision to have surgery. Reversely, interpreting, as do some of my acquaintances, my desire for a surgery as simply a refusal of ageing, doesn't do justice to the fact that in this case, maintaining a younger appearance is strongly linked to the expression of my gender identity (Siverskog, 2015, p 12). We can wonder: is my desire for a firm and flat chest anchored in gender dysphoria or 'ageing dysphoria'? In fact, it is not (just) gender dysphoria, nor is it (just) ageing dysphoria. This is trans ageing in action, in a messy and complex entanglement and continuous process. Indeed, while trans studies often puts the emphasis on the fact that transitions are ongoing processes rather than singular events in trans people's lives, the ageing process contributes to illuminating this reality. What I naïvely thought was a 'completed transition' has now become, with ageing, an ongoing transition process.

Moreover, the fact that one surgeon I consulted in a private clinic told me that he doesn't require a letter from a therapist to perform surgery since I am a "well-articulated, educated, intelligent and rational man" demonstrates how my Whiteness, class, education and cognitive ability play a key role in accessing healthcare, by removing some requirements imposed on others who do not have those privileges. The process would have been very different if I had revealed my mental illnesses or if I had a cognitive disability in our ableist/sanist/cogniticist contexts (Baril and Silverman, 2019; Silverman and Baril, 2021).[4] Additionally, education, class and financial privilege are inseparable from my age: the fact that I am now a tenured professor with a salary that allowed me to 'dress to impress' when I went to those clinics also made a difference. In sum, intersectional analyses are crucial to understanding these deep entanglements. Adopting an intersectional perspective to conceptualise the complex relationships between transness and ageing, and cisgenderism and ageism, helps us go beyond reductive interpretations of realities, situations, behaviours and discourses that consider transness and age as discrete ontological realities. These intersectional approaches, as Black feminist have shown in relation to Black women (Crenshaw, 1989; Hill Collins, 2000), are crucial for academics, practitioners and healthcare professionals if they want to better serve marginalised populations.

In conclusion, through an autoethnographic methodology using the examples of my corporeal changes that come with ageing – such as transformation in skin texture/elasticity or fat distribution – I focused in this chapter on my desire for top surgery. As previously discussed, while cisgender aging men face a delegitimisation of their masculinity as a result of ageist, ableist and heterosexist tropes associating 'real masculinity' with virility, ability and youth, this phenomenon takes a particular toll on middle-aged and older trans men who see their bodies changing with ageing, hence the importance for healthcare professionals and practitioners to abandon a silo mentality and to embrace an intersectional approach to trans health and ageing.

In closing, I would like to revisit the "Hey girls!" incident. Ellis et al (2011, np) argue that autoethnography is therapeutic not only for the authors but also for some readers who share the author's lived experience: 'Writing personal stories thus makes "witnessing" possible … As witnesses, autoethnographers … allow participants and readers to feel validated and/or better able to cope with or want to change their circumstances.' In other words, autoethnography aids autoethnographers and readers heal from various trauma. This chapter aims to offer other middle-aged or older trans people stories and conceptual tools to make sense of their own experiences and to validate their lived experiences. Writing this chapter also offered me a space to reflect on the difficult choice I am about to make regarding this surgery, and to gain a sense of healing from the incidents of intersecting ageist and cisgenderist violence I encounter in my daily life that find their ways into my own sense of embodiment.

"Hey girls!" are the two words that epitomise the beginning of my quest for a top surgery. As a proud feminist who graduated in feminist and gender studies, the girl/woman categories were always, and still are, so precious to me. Girlhood and womanhood have evoked a sense of pride, empowerment and political commitment. However, in the context of my transition towards masculinity, and the cisgenderist context in which I live, having this woman identity applied to me by a co-worker became enmeshed with a sense of shame. This chapter is an attempt to strike back and affirm my masculine identity in a cisgenderist and ageist world that invalidates it every day, and even more so the older I get. Repeating those two words, 'Hey girls!', is also an attempt to subvert, reclaim and remove the sense of shame associated with them ... Hey girls, hey boys and everyone in between, above and beyond those categories, do you want to join me in the fight for greater social justice? Let's not underestimate the power and strength of all those oldies trans folks who have been through hell to affirm proudly who they are today.

Summary learning points

- Provide critical reflections to better support ageing trans individuals.
- Offer concrete examples to better understand trans ageing through an autoethnographic account that centres on the lived experience of the author, who self-identifies as a trans disabled/Mad bisexual middle-aged man.
- Encourage dialogue between various fields of knowledge and intervention, such as those focusing on ageing populations, trans populations and men.
- Propose an intersectional analysis of the complex relationship between transness and age, and cisgenderism and ageism, which would be useful for understanding how older trans people experience social oppressions in different ways.

Notes

[1] Arguments in this chapter have been presented in: Baril, A. 'Trans(ition) time: Transgender subjectivities and the aging masculine body,' 47th British Society of Gerontology Conference, University of Manchester, 6 July 2018.

[2] I employ the capitalised term 'Mad' to denote the resignified positive label embraced by individuals who have experienced psychiatric treatment, survivors former patients or users of mental health services, reclaiming their experiences of madness. This terminology is commonly utilised within the field of Mad studies, by scholars specialising in this area, and by those who identify with the Mad movement.

[3] For genealogies and definitions of 'cisgenderism' and 'cisnormativity', see Silverman and Baril (2021).

[4] For a definition of cogniticism, see Silverman and Baril (2021).

References

Ansara, Y.G. (2015) 'Challenging cisgenderism in the ageing and aged care sector: meeting the needs of older people of trans and/or non-binary experience', *Australasian Journal on Ageing*, 34: 14–18.

Bailey, L. (2012) 'Trans ageing: thoughts on a life course approach in order to better understand trans lives', in R. Ward, M. Sutherland and I. Rivers (eds) *Lesbian, Gay, Bisexual and Transgender Ageing: Biographical Approaches for Inclusive Care and Support*, London: Jessica Kingsley Publishers, pp 30–8.

Bailey, L., McNeil, J. and Ellis, S.J. (2019) 'Mental health and well-being among older trans people', in A. King, K. Almack, Y.-T. Suen and S. Westwood (eds) *Older Lesbian, Gay, Bisexual and Trans People: Minding the Knowledge Gaps*, London: Routledge, pp 44–60.

Baril, A. and Silverman, M. (2019) 'Forgotten lives: trans older adults living with dementia at the intersection of cisgenderism, ableism/cogniticism and ageism', *Sexualities* [online]: 1–15. DOI: 10.1177/1363460719876835.

Benbow, S.M., Eost-Telling, C. and Kingston, P. (2022) 'A narrative review of literature on the use of health and social care by older trans adults: what can United Kingdom services learn?', *Ageing & Society*, 42(10): 2262–83.

Bishop, J.-A. and Westwood, S. (2019) 'Trans(gender)/gender-diverse ageing', in S. Westwood (ed) *Ageing, Diversity and Equality: Social Justice Perspectives*, London: Routledge, pp 82–97.

Cook-Daniels, L. (2015) 'Transgender ageing: what practitioners should know', in N.A. Orel and C.A. Fruhauf (eds) *The Lives of LGBT Older Adults*, Washington, DC: American Psychological Association, pp 193–215.

Crenshaw, K. (1989) 'Demarginalizing the intersection of race and sex: a Black feminist critique of discrimination doctrine, feminist theory and antiracist practice', *University of Chicago Legal Forum*, 1989(1): 139–67.

Dubois, L.Z., SturtzSreetharan, C., MacFife, B., Puckett, J.A., Jagielski, A., Dunn, T.A. et al (2022) 'Trans and gender diverse people's experience wearing face masks during the COVID-19 pandemic: findings from data across 4 states in the USA', *Sexuality Research and Social Policy*: 1–9 [online], Available from: https:// DOI: 10.1007/s13178-022-00781-0.

Ellis, C., Adams, T.E. and Bochner, A.P. (2011) 'Autoethnography: an overview', *Qualitative Social Research*, 12(1), [online], Available from: http://nbn-resolving.de/urn:nbn:de:0114-fqs1101108

Fabbre, V.D. (2014) 'Gender transitions in later life: the significance of time in queer aging', *Journal of Gerontological Social Work*, 57(2–4): 161–75.

Fabbre, V.D. and Gaveras, E. (2020) 'The manifestation of multilevel stigma in the lived experiences of transgender and gender nonconforming older adults', *American Journal of Orthopsychiatry*, 90(3): 350–60.

Fabbre, V.D. and Siverskog, A. (2020) 'Transgender ageing: community resistance and well-being in the life course', in A. King, K. Almack and R.L. Jones (eds) *Intersections of Ageing, Gender and Sexualities: Multidisciplinary International Perspectives*, Bristol: Policy Press, pp 47–62.

Fredriksen-Goldsen, K., Cook-Daniels, L., Kim, H.J., Erosheva, E.A., Emlet, C.A., Hoy-Ellis, C.P. et al (2014) 'Physical and mental health of transgender older adults: an at-risk and underserved population', *The Gerontologist*, 54(3): 488–500.

Hardacker, C., Ducheny, K. and Houlberg, M. (eds) (2019) *Transgender and Gender Nonconforming Health and Aging*, Cham: Springer.

Hébert, W., Enriquez, M.C. and Chamberland, L. (2013) 'Working with trans elders: finding the resources to make the health and social services sectors more inclusive', unpublished report.

Hill Collins, P. (2000) *Black Feminist Thought: Knowledge, Consciousness, and the Politics of Empowerment* (2nd edn), New York: Routledge.

Holzmer, S.W., Lewis, P.G., Landau, M.J. and Hill, M.E. (2020) 'Surgical management of gynecomastia: a comprehensive review of the literature', *Plastic and Reconstructive Surgery Global Open*, 8(10): e3161. DOI: 10.1097/GOX.0000000000003161

Latham, J.R. and Barrett, C. (2015) 'Trans health and ageing: an evidence-based guide to inclusive services', Melbourne: La Trobe University.

Nowakowski, A.C.H., Sumerau, J.E. and Mathers, L.A.B. (2021) 'Health and ageing among middle and later age transgender populations', in A.H. Johnson, B.A. Rogers and T. Taylor (eds) *Advances in Trans Studies: Moving toward Gender Expansion and Trans Hope*, Bingley: Emerald Publishing Limited, pp 9–27.

Pang, C., Gutman, G. and de Vries, B. (2019) 'Later life care planning and concerns of transgender older adults in Canada', *The International Journal of Aging and Human Development*, 89(1): 39–56.

Pearce, R. (2019) 'Trans temporalities and non-linear ageing', in A. King, K. Almack, Y.-T. Suen and S. Westwood (eds) *Older Lesbian, Gay, Bisexual and Trans People: Minding the Knowledge Gaps*, London: Routledge, pp 61–74.

Porter, K.E., Brennan-Ing, M., Chang, S.C., Dickey, L.M., Singh, A.A., Bower, K.L. et al (2016) 'Providing competent and affirming services for transgender and gender nonconforming older adults', *Clinical Gerontologist*, 39(5): 366–88.

Serano, J. (2007) *Whipping Girl: A Transsexual Woman on Sexism and the Scapegoating of Femininity*, Berkeley: Seal Press.

Silverman, M. and Baril, A. (2021) 'Transing dementia: rethinking compulsory biographical continuity through the theorization of cisism and cisnormativity', *Journal of Aging Studies*, 58: 1–9.

Silverman, M. and Baril, A. (2023) '"We have to advocate so hard for ourselves and our people": caring for a trans or non-binary older adult with dementia', *LGBTQ+ Family: An Interdisciplinary Journal*, 19(3): 187–210. DOI: 10.1080/27703371.2023.2169215

Siverskog, A. (2014) '"They just don't have a clue": transgender aging and implications for social work', *Journal of Gerontological Social Work*, 57(2–4): 386–406.

Siverskog, A. (2015) 'Ageing bodies that matter: age, gender and embodiment in older transgender people's life stories', *NORA: Nordic Journal of Feminist and Gender Research*, 23(1): 4–19.

Toze, M. (2019) 'Developing a critical trans gerontology', *British Journal of Sociology*, 70(4): 1490–509.

Toze, M. (2021) 'Invisible futures: trans men and representations of ageing', *Intersectional Perspectives: Identity, Culture, and Society*, 1: 53–73.

White, F.R. (2014) 'Fat/trans: queering the activist body', *Fat Studies: An Interdisciplinary Journal of Body Weight and Society*, 3(2): 86–100.

Willis, P., Raithby, M., Dobbs, C., Evans, E. and Bishop, J.-A. (2021) '"I'm going to live my life for me": trans ageing, care, and older trans and gender non-conforming adults' expectations of and concerns for later life', *Ageing & Society*, 41(12): 2792–813.

Witten, T.M. (2003) 'Life course analysis: the courage to search for something more; middle adulthood issues in the transgender and intersex community', in M.K. Sullivan (ed) *Sexual Minorities: Discrimination, Challenges, and Development in America*, New York: Haworth Press, pp 189–224.

Witten, T.M. and Eyler, A.E. (2012) 'Transgender and aging: beings and becoming', in T.M. Witten and A.E. Eyler (eds) *Gay, Lesbian, Bisexual and Transgender Aging: Challenges in Research, Practice and Policy*, Baltimore: Johns Hopkins University Press, pp 187–269.

6

Examining the views and attitudes of health and social care professionals towards older trans people: findings from the Trans Ageing and Care study

Deborah Morgan, Paul Willis and Christine Dobbs

Introduction

In this chapter, we focus on the perceptions and attitudes of health and social care professionals towards older trans people in the United Kingdom. Within the UK, the need for systemic change in delivering inclusive healthcare for trans people is a longstanding issue. In 2016, the UK House of Commons Women and Equalities Committee identified significant problems in delivering good standards of care to trans individuals accessing trans-related healthcare, including professionals' knowledge levels and trans people's experiences of discriminatory treatment. In 2019, the Royal College of General Practitioners called for a whole-system approach to improving services for trans patients. More recent research on integrated care for trans adults has highlighted persistent gaps in professional knowledge levels and service provision (inclusive of GPs), leading to a renewed call for developing more person-led models of gender-affirming care (Holti et al, 2023).

It is important to acknowledge that not all trans individuals wish to access gender-affirming treatments or transition through surgical and/or medical means; regardless, they will have contact with helping professionals regarding other health and social care needs. Indeed, large survey findings show that there is likely to be an increase in the number of people from younger generations identifying as gender non-conforming and therefore being less likely to identify as trans as they age in the UK (Government Equalities Office, 2018). The same survey has highlighted that UK trans citizens report lower levels of life satisfaction compared to LGB and non-LGB cisgender people and experience multiple barriers to healthcare, including having their specific needs ignored and being the subject of inappropriate questions (Government Equalities Office, 2018). There is much work to be done in moving towards a trans-inclusive approach to health and social care delivery for people with care and support needs, including those in later life. This is even more imperative in the context of an ageing population with predicted higher numbers of trans citizens needing access to good housing, health and social care services to support their wellbeing, rights and dignity in later life. Gaining a deeper understanding of how health and social care professionals perceive and make sense of trans people's care and support needs in later life is one part of developing a good evidence base to trigger systemic change.

In this chapter, we present and discuss survey findings from the 'Trans Ageing and Care' (TrAC) study (2016–19)[1] that have not been published elsewhere. This mixed-methods study aimed to generate new evidence about the care and support needs of trans people entering later life in Wales. A total of 165 health and social care professionals across Wales completed an online questionnaire that assessed respondents' knowledge about trans' legal and medical issues in later life, familiarity with trans individuals, levels of support for trans civil rights and beliefs about gender diversity and trans issues. Findings indicate respondents are trans aware and familiar with trans issues (with the media being the most popular source) and are generally supportive of trans civil rights. However, there were identified gaps in respondents' knowledge about trans issues in later life (medical and legal knowledge) and a call for more education and training. We conclude by outlining four core components essential to developing a trans-inclusive training curriculum that takes into account the needs of trans individuals in later life.

Background to the study

Previously published findings from the TrAC study highlighted the obstacles and discrimination trans people in mid to later life encounter when seeking to access gender identity services (Willis et al, 2020, 2021). These include long delays in trans individuals receiving clinic referrals and accessing services, uncertainty about the future coupled with a sense of 'running out of time', the need to self-advocate and educate GPs about available services and healthcare entitlements, and the logistical challenges in accessing gender-affirming treatments and assessment services that were more often a considerable distance from home. Similar barriers and challenges have been identified in other UK studies, highlighting processes for accessing gender-affirming treatments as complicated to navigate (Holti et al, 2023; Mill et al, 2023).

Studies of other professional groups indicate heterogeneity in views and attitudes towards working with trans individuals and groups. Survey findings from a study of Australian mental health professionals suggest a positive correlation between contact with trans individuals and training received and increased confidence in providing support to trans patients.

The same study highlights a negative relationship between religiosity and levels of comfort in supporting trans people (Riggs and Bartholomaeus, 2016). In the UK, a survey of therapists indicates that these professionals generally hold positive attitudes towards trans people but are hindered by anxieties about 'getting it wrong' when delivering therapeutic support and using incorrect words and terminology. A minority of therapists report transphobic views and continue to frame trans identity as a 'psychological illness' (being trans is not classified as a mental disorder or illness under current diagnostic manuals or international classifications) (Mollitt, 2022). Mollitt's findings contain a small minority of therapists disagreeing with a legal ban on conversion therapies. This is particularly alarming given that many older trans people will have been offered or referred for conversion therapy in earlier decades when disclosing trans subjectivities to healthcare professionals. Qualitative research on social workers' views and attitudes suggests that, while social workers in Sweden remain committed to principles of equal treatment, normative discourses about gender and sexuality get in the way of providing trans-inclusive practice (Smolle and Espvall, 2021). In the TrAC study, we focused on the views and attitudes of health and social care professionals to get a better understanding of how trans patients and clients may be received and treated by practitioners and what the gaps are in thinking about future training needs.

Brief note about the survey design and respondents

We created an online questionnaire to assess professionals' knowledge about trans legal and medical issues in later life, familiarity with trans individuals, levels of support for trans civil rights and beliefs about gender diversity and trans issues. Data for the online questionnaire were collected between 2017 and 2018, and several validated scales and composite measures were used. Validated measures included the levels of support for 'Trans Civil Rights' sub-scale (six items adapted from Tee and Hegarty, 2006), and 'Beliefs about Transexuality' sub-scale (authors' terminology) (12 items adapted from Tee and Hegarty, 2006). Demographic variables included: current age; gender (male/female/other); gender history; sexual orientation; current relationship status; job title, length of time in current role and highest professional qualification; place of birth; ethnic background; and faith group or beliefs. Other items are reported subsequently. All respondents gave informed consent before proceeding to questionnaire items. At the end of the questionnaire, respondents had the option of entering a prize draw to win four £50 high-street store vouchers and were given access to contact details for additional support services, including Wales-based trans organisations and groups. The questionnaire and accompanying information about taking part, including flyers, were provided bilingually in line with Welsh language requirements.

Links and information about the survey were circulated through a number of channels: equality leads across health boards (in charge of coordinating and commissioning healthcare services in local areas); service managers for all local authority adult services in Wales; mail outs and newsletters targeted at different professional groups (including GPs and social workers); and through regulatory professional bodies, for example Social Care Wales. The survey was open for 12 months to maximise responses. The sample is non-representative, as it was not possible to build a sampling framework, and it is likely that the questionnaire attracted individuals who were already trans-supportive (but not in all cases, as one respondent conveyed discriminatory views in their open-ended responses about trans people being 'undeserving' of NHS services). Consequently, the findings give a flavour of professionals' views and attitudes and cannot be generalised to wider professional groups. Nonetheless, this is a valuable contribution to a limited knowledge base on professionals' views and attitudes.

A total of 165 health and social care professionals completed the survey. Respondents worked in a variety of professional roles, with just over half (50.3 per cent) working in healthcare roles (GPs, clinicians, mental health staff), while just over a quarter of respondents (25.5 per cent) identified as having a healthcare management or administrative role, and 20 per cent of respondents identified as working in social care or social work. Most of the respondents (62 per cent) had been in their role for less than ten years. The sample was predominantly White (93 per cent), female (77.6 per cent) and originating from the UK (91 per cent). Only 20 per cent of respondents identified as male, and just 1.8 per cent identified as other. Likewise, most of the sample identified as heterosexual (84.2 per cent), with 8 per cent of respondents self-identifying as gay/lesbian, 3.6 per cent as bisexual and 0.6 per cent identifying as queer. Regarding the age of the sample, 51 per cent of respondents were under 45 years old.

What did we find? Ascertaining gaps in professionals' knowledge

The survey findings demonstrate that respondents were trans-aware and appeared to be generally supportive of trans rights and access to gender-affirming treatments. However, the findings also revealed significant gaps and variations in knowledge. Variations in knowledge were identified in relation to familiarity with trans issues, in the knowledge of trans issues and in confidence levels for working with trans people. Taking each in turn, variations and gaps in knowledge will be highlighted and discussed, beginning with respondents' familiarity with trans issues.

Familiarity with trans people and issues

The five familiarity items in the questionnaire assessed whether respondents were familiar with and had exposure to trans issues. These were taken with permission from a survey developed by Riggs and Bartholomaeus (2016). These included questions relating to (1) whether respondents had read information on the controversy over gender dysphoria as a formal diagnosis (now referred to as gender incongruence by the World Health Organization), (2) met someone who identifies as transgender, (3) read information in the media about transgender people, (4) read information regarding presenting issues common to older adults and (5) whether they have a friend or family member who identifies as transgender. Response options for these questions were yes/no.

The findings show that just over half of the respondents (55.8 per cent) were aware of and had read information on the controversy over gender dysphoria as a formal diagnosis. However, less was known about presenting issues that are common among trans older adults, with only 59 respondents (36 per cent) indicating that they had read information about specific issues among older trans people. What was evident is that the media was a popular source of information, with 90 per cent of respondents reading information about trans people in the media. With regard to whether respondents had met someone outside of their professional role who identified as trans, two thirds of respondents (65.5 per cent) said they had met someone who identified as trans, with 19 per cent responding they had a friend or family member who identified as transgender.

Ascertaining confidence in working with trans clients

Another variable of interest was the variations in the 'Confidence in Working with Trans Clients Measure' (also from Riggs and Bartholomaeus, 2016). This measure assessed health and social care professionals' confidence in their ability to provide a service for transgender people (term 'transgender' used in the scale). This scale originally comprised six items. For the purpose of our survey, we adopted the following four items: (1) I feel confident in providing a health or social care service to older (50+) transgender adults, (2) I feel confident in providing a health or social care service to younger transgender adults, (3) I feel confident in providing a health or social care service to transgender children and adolescents, (4) I feel confident in providing a health or social care service to friends and family of older (50+) transgender adults. Responses were on a five-point Likert scale ranging from not at all confident, somewhat lacking in confidence, neither confident nor lacking in confidence, somewhat confident through to very confident. The original scale produced by Riggs and Bartholomaeus (2016) referred to 'mental health services' – this was changed to 'health or social care service' in line with the aims of the TrAC study. Two items that referred to providing a mental health service to parents of transgender people and parents of transgender children were dropped as again these did not align with the study aims.

Our analysis shows that 60 per cent of respondents felt somewhat confident or very confident in providing a service to trans older adults, with 19 per cent responding they were somewhat lacking in confidence or not confident. The findings were similar to the question regarding confidence in providing a service to younger transgender adults, with just over half of respondents (57 per cent) indicating they were somewhat confident or very confident. Likewise, 61 per cent of respondents felt confident in providing a health or social care service to friends and family of older transgender adults, with just 3 per cent not being confident and 14 per cent somewhat lacking confidence. However, in contrast, fewer respondents felt confident in providing a health and social care service to children and adolescents, with 17 per cent stating not confident and 27 per cent somewhat lacking in confidence. Just a third of respondents felt confident or somewhat confident in providing a service to this cohort.

Assessing knowledge about trans issues in later life

The research team designed 11 statements to assess respondents' knowledge of key legal and medical requirements and issues associated with accessing gender-affirming treatments, gaining formal recognition of gender and issues associated with later life. Response options were true/false/don't know. Responses were then coded as correct, incorrect and don't know, with some statements being correct if the response to a statement was false while other statements were correct if the response to the statement was true (see Table 6.1). These statements were developed through consultation with the project's critical reference group and were based on information outlined in the Age UK (2015) factsheet 'Transgender issues in later life'. In addition, we consulted a general practitioner with recognised expertise in supporting trans individuals on the accuracy of medical-related statements.

Although it was clear that respondents had some knowledge of trans issues, there remained significant gaps and variations in their knowledge relating to key issues facing trans people. Indeed, while some statements were correctly identified as true/false by most respondents, other statements were incorrectly identified by the majority of the respondents, while responses to two of the statements presented were predominantly 'don't know'. We discuss these subsequently, beginning with statements that respondents correctly identified as true or false.

In total, five statements were answered correctly by over 60 per cent of respondents. These included responses to the statement: *things like retirement*

Table 6.1: Statements assessing respondents' knowledge of key legal and medical requirements

1. A transgender person must end their marriage before they can change their legal identity.
2. Things like retirement from work or the death of a partner could provide the trigger to allow a person to think about and act upon their desire to transition.
3. In Wales, an in-depth assessment must be carried out by at least two specialists before any older person considering transitioning can have access to any form of treatment.
4. Before any gender surgery can be given, the person wishing this must have lived in their preferred gender role for at least 12 months.
5. The Gender Recognition Act 2004 has made it possible for a transgender person to apply for a Gender Recognition Certificate.
6. If a person in their professional capacity has learnt that an individual has a Gender Recognition Certificate, they may share this information without that individual's permission.
7. The Equality Act 2010 does not protect those *intending* to live permanently in their preferred gender role.
8. The reporting of transgender hate crime has risen year on year since 2011.
9. Currently, obtaining a Gender Recognition Certificate can affect things such as pension benefits.
10. Irrespective of whether a birth relative is still alive or not, a transgender person's unrelated significant other without Power of Attorney can register their death.
11. When a transgender person without a Gender Recognition Certificate dies, their death certificate is issued in their birth identity.

Note: Here and elsewhere in the questionnaire, the term 'transgender' was used as an umbrella term inclusive of people identifying as trans (including those seeking to access gender-affirming treatments), non-binary and gender non-conforming. This term was agreed with the project's critical reference group of which over half the membership identified as trans. A definition of this term was provided to respondents at the commencement of the questionnaire.

from work or a partner's death could trigger a person to think about and act upon their desire to transition, with 74 per cent of respondents answering that this was true. Similarly, most respondents (77.6 per cent) were aware that individuals wishing to have gender surgery *must have lived in their preferred gender role for at least 12 months*, and 20 per cent of the respondents responded as not knowing whether this was a true or false statement. At the same time, 60 per cent of respondents were aware that the Gender Recognition Act 2004 enabled a transgender person to apply for a Gender Recognition Certificate (this currently applies across the UK). Likewise, 77.6 per cent of respondents were aware that in their professional roles, they could not share information that an individual has a Gender Recognition Certificate without that person's explicit permission; only one person responded incorrectly to this statement, while the remainder stated that they didn't know. Finally, 72.7 per cent of respondents knew that reported hate crimes against transgender people had increased since 2011.

In contrast, two statements elicited responses suggesting that knowledge of these among some health and social care professionals was lacking. In response to the statement relating to whether a transgender person must end their marriage before they can legally change their identity, 58.2 per cent correctly responded that this statement was false; however, 32 per cent of respondents didn't know, and 9.7 per cent responded incorrectly that this was a true statement. It is worth noting that this statement used to be true – so some respondents who responded incorrectly may be relying on outdated information. Similarly, 40 per cent of respondents didn't know that an older person considering transitioning in Wales must have an in-depth assessment by two specialists before they can access treatment, while 7.3 per cent incorrectly responded that this statement was false.

Finally, four statements elicited incorrect responses from most respondents. In response to the statement *the Equality Act 2010 does not protect those intending to live permanently in their preferred gender role*, 60 per cent of respondents either responded they didn't know (47.9 per cent) or incorrectly identified the statement as true (12.7 per cent). Only 39 per cent correctly responded that the statement was false. Likewise, most respondents were unaware that obtaining a Gender Recognition Certificate could affect things such as a person's pension benefits, with 66 per cent not knowing whether this statement was true or false and 12.7 per cent responding that this was false. There was also a lack of knowledge about whether an unrelated significant other without Power of Attorney could register the death of a transgender person, with only 20.6 per cent of respondents correctly identifying this statement to be false. Most respondents either did not know the correct response (69.7 per cent) or incorrectly responded that this statement was true (9.7 per cent). Finally, half of the respondents to the survey were unaware that if a transgender person dies without a Gender Recognition Certificate, their death certificate is issued in their birth identity (we note that this issue is currently the subject of legal debate in the UK and as such not entirely clear in law). Whereas 82 respondents (49.7 per cent) correctly identified this statement as true, 44.2 per cent responded that they did not know and 6.1 per cent incorrectly responded that the statement was true. More knowledge and clarity is needed on this key legal issue that could severely impact recognition for an older trans person's wishes at end of life or autonomy if they were to experience a decline in cognitive capacity, for example a dementia-related illness.

It is evident from these responses that while health and social care professionals have some knowledge of trans issues, there are also notable gaps in knowledge. These are particularly evident around issues such as the Equality Act 2010 (under which 'gender reassignment' is a protected characteristic), the lack of awareness around the implications to pension rights resulting from obtaining a Gender Recognition Certificate and who can register the death of a trans person. Furthermore, there is also a lack of knowledge about the rights of trans people, specifically concerning the right to remain married when someone wishes to legally change their identity but also around the need for in-depth assessments for older people wishing to transition. There was no evidence in the data that factors such as respondents' age, ethnicity, gender, sexual orientation, religion, location or job had a significant role in their familiarity or knowledge of transgender issues or their confidence in working with trans people within their service.

Accessing training and professional development activities

What is evident from the findings is the need for enhancing pre- and post-qualifying training and education for health and social care professionals. This is important because the variations in knowledge about trans people translate as variations in the care and services provided by different health and social care professionals. Regarding continuing professional development, we asked respondents about their experiences of training on gender identity and trans-related support to date. This is critical to explore in the context that training received on trans awareness is a predictor of increased confidence and comfort levels among helping professionals (Riggs and Bartholomaeus, 2016). Over two thirds of respondents (116) indicated they had received no training in working with trans clients or patients, with a small number expressing a wish for this. A total of 27 respondents reported receiving some training in this area – this varied from half-day sessions with trans speakers through to reading online or completion of online modules on gender identity issues provided by the Royal College of General Practitioners (for GP respondents). In the main, training was referred to as a single session with some involvement of trans speakers. Well over half of the respondents (100) indicated a need for further education, training and knowledge enhancement, with at least a third of these respondents emphasising the importance of hearing a trans person's story or personal experience first hand. Increased knowledge about legal issues was repeatedly requested; this tallies with the findings showing variations and gaps in respondents' knowledge of key legal issues associated with older age.

These findings are encouraging in the sense that *some* training is being delivered and received, and, in some instances, this has been delivered by and with trans citizens. We favour a co-designed model of training with trans individuals and groups where the voices of trans citizens are central to the delivery of training and key information. Based on the responses, it would seem our respondents also have an appetite for more direct contact with and first-hand accounts from trans people. However, the involvement of trans individuals in training and professional education needs to be sufficiently resourced through continuous support and supervision and appropriate remuneration. Our earlier findings highlight the burden of educating other professionals, particularly GPs, which often falls on the shoulders of trans people in mid to later life when seeking to access gender-affirming treatments (see Willis et al, 2000). Another note of caution is that hearing a trans person's personal account is not the same as receiving comprehensive training, but it may be a useful starting point or helpful element of training.

Conclusion: moving towards a trans-inclusive curriculum

There have been a number of significant shifts and changes in the social and political landscape of the UK since we ran the TrAC survey. Here we reflect on how these may impact on professionals' attitudes before discussing the imperative to develop trans-inclusive curriculums for professionals. First, since we ran the survey Wales has established its own Welsh Gender Service (NHS Wales, nd), and at the heart of this model is the delivery of local gender teams made up of GPs and speech and language therapists. It is reasonable to expect that the creation of these local teams will help improve healthcare professionals' knowledge more broadly, at least at a primary care level. More evidence is needed to determine this. Second, at an international level, new 'Standards of care for the health of transgender and gender diverse people' have been published by the World Professional Association for Transgender Health (Coleman et al, 2022). These are clinical guidelines and principles which clearly state that gender-affirming care applies to trans people 'across the lifespan – from the very first signs of gender incongruence in childhood through adulthood and into older age' (p 57). Third, there has been increased negative publicity surrounding trans people and political debates about 'trans rights' in recent years. This follows UK government proposals in 2017 to reform the Gender Recognition Act 2004 and give trans people the right to self-determine their gender (proposals now scrapped by the current Sunak Government) (Pearce et al, 2020). In parallel, the political backlash against trans people and groups has been amplified in the news and on social media, so much so that at the time of writing this chapter a United Nations Independent Expert (2023) has commented on 'widespread concerns over toxic political discourse' (p 5) in the UK and accompanying transphobic rhetoric conveyed through the media. This is concerning given that most of our survey respondents look to the news media as a key source of information. A further observation is that current media attention on trans issues is often focused on children and younger people, which contributes to the invisibility of older trans people in the public sphere. Trans older people will have lived through many decades of exclusionary and restricted media representation about trans' lives, and the long-term impact on people's sense of self-worth needs to be a critical consideration in supporting older adults. This acutely sharpens the need for developing alternative evidence-based sources that are reliable, trans affirming and accessible for health and social care professionals. Other researchers have established that experience in working with trans individuals and training related to this are two predictors of increased confidence among helping professionals (Riggs and Bartholomaeus, 2016).

Based on our findings, we argue that the following four components are essential for developing a trans-inclusive curriculum that takes into account the needs of trans individuals in later life. The first component is the supported involvement of older trans individuals in training design and delivery – this may be in the form of co-designed and co-delivered sessions but will depend on the capacity for trans individuals to be involved; their involvement should not be onerous or rest solely on their shoulders. We argue this based on the importance of professionals having direct conversations and first-hand contact with trans individuals and the way in which this can sharpen their receptiveness to trans people's experiences and perspectives across the life course. The second component is about enhancing legal literacy among professionals within a rights-based framework, particularly around legal issues pertinent to older age and end of life. The third component is providing professionals with some basic medical knowledge that counteracts ageist assumptions that older people are 'too old' to receive gender-affirming treatments and that instead highlights that there are options available to trans people in later life. This includes avoiding assumptions that all trans people wish to transition in later life. The fourth and final component is the importance of adopting a life course perspective to recognise and understand how anticipated discrimination, social stigma and cisnormative arrangements experienced over many decades can impair people's trust and confidence in health and social care professionals in old age. Central to any training delivery is the recognition that practitioners have a professional responsibility to create safe and affirming environments across housing, health and social care services and to ensure this is clearly articulated to trans people from first point of contact with their services.

Summary learning points

- Gaps exist in health and social care professionals' knowledge about legal rights for older trans people, and there is a demand from professionals for more training and skills provision in supporting trans clients and patients.
- The media is a popular source of information for professionals and brings with it the risk of misleading and toxic information about trans' lives and identities.
- Direct contact with trans individuals and hearing first-hand accounts about their lived experiences is a critical component for developing

future training and continuing professional development activities. But it shouldn't be the only component of training.
- Training and continuing professional development activities require a focus on developing legal literacy for promoting older trans people's rights and should contain content that counteracts ageist assumptions about transitioning in later life.

Note

[1] The TraC study was hosted by the Centre for Innovative Ageing at Swansea University in collaboration with the University of Bristol. The study received ethical approval from the College of Human and Health Sciences Research Ethics Committee, Swansea University (2016).

References

Coleman, E., Bouman, W.P., Brown, G.R., de Vries, A.L.C., Deutsch, M.B., Ettner, R. et al (2022) 'Standards of care for the health of transgender and gender diverse people, version 8', *International Journal of Transgender Health*, 23(sup1): S1–S259.

Government Equalities Office (2018) 'National LGBT survey: summary report', London: UK government, [online], Available from: https://www.gov.uk/government/publications/national-lgbt-survey-summary-report

Holti, R., Callaghan, E., Fletcher, J., Hope, S., Moller, N., Vincent, B. et al (2023) 'Improving the integration of care for trans adults (ICTA): final report of a project funded by the National Institute for Health and Care Research (NIHR) (HSDR 17/51/08)', Milton Keynes: Open University.

Mills, T.J., Riddell, K.E., Price, E. and Smith, D.R.R. (2023) '"Stuck in the system": an interpretative phenomenological analysis of transmasculine experiences of gender transition in the UK', *Qualitative Health Research*, [online], 5 April, 33(7): 57–88, Available from: https://doi.org/10.1177/10497323231167779

Mollitt, P.C. (2022) 'Exploring cisgender therapists' attitudes towards, and experience of, working with trans people in the United Kingdom', *Counselling and Psychotherapy Research*, 22(4): 1013–29.

NHS Wales (nd) 'Welsh Gender Service', [online], Available from: https://cavuhb.nhs.wales/our-services/welsh-gender-service/

Pearce, R., Erikainen, S. and Vincent, B. (2020) 'TERF wars: an introduction', *The Sociological Review Monographs*, 68(4): 677–98.

Riggs, D.W. and Bartholomaeus, C. (2016) 'Australian mental health professionals' competencies for working with trans clients: a comparative study', *Psychology and Sexuality*, 7(3): 225–38.

Smolle, S. and Espvall, M. (2021) 'Transgender competence in social work with older adults in Sweden', *Journal of Social Service Research*, 47(4): 522–36.

Tee, N. and Hegarty, P. (2006) 'Predicting opposition to the civil rights of trans persons in the United Kingdom', *Journal of Community and Applied Social Psychology*, 16(1): 70–80.

United Nations (2023) 'United Nations independent expert on protection against violence and discrimination based on sexual orientation and gender identity: country visit to the United Kingdom of Great Britain and Northern Ireland (24 April–5 May 2023)', [online], Available from: https://www.ohchr.org/sites/default/files/documents/issues/sexualorientation/statements/eom-statement-UK-IE-SOGI-2023-05-10.pdf

Willis, P., Dobbs, C., Evans, E., Raithby, M. and Bishop, J-A. (2020) 'Reluctant educators and self-advocates: older trans adults' experiences of healthcare services and practitioners in seeking gender affirming services', *Health Expectations*, 23(5): 1231–40.

Willis, P., Raithby, M., Dobbs, C., Evans, E. and Bishop, J.-A. (2021) '"I'm going to live my life for me": trans ageing, care and older trans and gender non-conforming adults' expectations of and concerns for later life', *Ageing and Society*, 41(12): 2792–813.

7

Professional preparedness for supporting older transgender adults when working in social services in Sweden

Sofia Smolle

Introduction

In 2020, the European Commission published the 'LGBTIQ equality strategy 2020–2025', which calls on member states to strengthen legal rights and protections for transgender people (as a part of the LGBTIQ umbrella term). The strategy involves dealing with discrimination against this part of the population, ensuring their direct safety as well as forming inclusive societies. The strategy is important given that it is reported that trans people experience substantial discrimination, vulnerabilities and internalised stigma. This seems to be especially true for older trans adults (Vincent and Velkoff, 2010; Fredriksen-Goldsen et al, 2013; Siverskog, 2016; SOU, 2017, p 92), who face a high risk of deteriorating health, mental illness and poverty (Grant et al, 2011; Fredriksen-Goldsen et al, 2013; Kattari et al, 2020).

Despite their vulnerability, research on this group of people in social work is limited. This holds true for many countries, including Sweden and other Nordic countries. In previous Swedish research, it has been shown that older trans adults fear becoming recipients of care as they grow older (Siverskog, 2014; Löf and Olaison, 2018). A specific fear is of being treated poorly by caregivers due to ignorance or a lack of knowledge about trans issues (Siverskog, 2014; SOU, 2017). Research also indicates a fear among caregivers in the form of professional insecurities when discussing future care for older trans adults (Smolle and Espvall, 2021). However, research on these issues remains limited. Thus the purpose of this study is to give examples of issues such as professional prerequisites and insecurities from the perspective of social workers (who to their knowledge have not yet provided professional services to older trans adults). The chapter focuses in particular on professional preparedness for supporting older trans adults among social workers in the municipal social services in Sweden.

The Swedish context

In Sweden, it is prohibited to discriminate against persons based on their gender identity and gender expression (Swedish Discrimination Act 2008). The law applies in several areas, for instance in working life, education, healthcare and municipal social services.

In Sweden, as in the other Nordic welfare states, social work is mainly carried out within municipality organisations. Municipal social work is specified and regulated in the Social Services Act 2001. In this law, older adults are included as an especially vulnerable group. For example, social services must prioritise the wellbeing of all older people. Thus, social services for older adults as well as healthcare for the group are parts of the Swedish welfare system. Unfortunately, several reports by Swedish authorities have highlighted that the LGBTQ rights are not prioritised within this system. This is especially the case concerning social services and care for older adults. It is also reported that LGBTQ people themselves have low trust in institutions, and this is especially low among trans people (Public Health Agency of Sweden, 2015; SOU, 2017). Research has also indicated that several welfare institutions that provide care and support are characterised by cisnormativity, which affects both caregivers and care seekers (Bremer, 2011; Linander et al, 2019; Smolle and Espvall, 2021). One example of this is when gender identity is assumed when meeting older adults in assessment or in a care situation. If not asked about or in other ways expressed, this might lead to 'trans' needs being accorded less importance (Smolle and Espvall, 2021). It has been shown that many social workers lack specific training in trans-affirmative support and norm-critical approaches within their social work education and/or organisational training. Also, cisnormativity is not questioned to a high degree because trans-related issues are not prioritised in the political fields or within municipal social work organisations (Smolle and Espvall, 2021). However, these issues have increasingly been on the agenda of Swedish authorities for the last 20 years, which is due to non-profit organisations (such as the Swedish Federation for Lesbian, Gay, Bisexual, Transgender, Queer and Intersex Rights) pushing these issues politically (Summanen, 2023). It is also mainly these organisations that offer further training to social workers and other care professionals in trans-related issues in order to increase trans-affirmative care and support.

The study

In this study (which is part of a more extensive project that was reviewed and approved by the Swedish Ethical Review Authority in Umeå in 2018, doc no 2018/261–31), I conducted qualitative interviews with 16 social workers working in municipal social services in Sweden. I initially made contact with managers and social workers within municipalities who forwarded information about the study to their colleagues. The social workers who thereafter reported an interest in participating were given information about the study. According to the participating social workers themselves, they had not, to their knowledge, had experiences of meeting or supporting older trans adults. The social workers were 25 to 65 years old, and they were all cisgender and straight, except for one person identifying as gay, who explained that although they had personal experience of trans people from being part of the LGBTQ community, they had no professional experience of working with members of this community. The majority had a degree in social work, and the rest had a university degree in another care-related subject, such as a nursing degree. Their work experience ranged from one to 20 years. Most of the participating social workers worked specifically with assessing the need for support and social care interventions for older adults. A few of them worked in a broader area within municipal social services, and they were consequently in a position to come into contact with older persons. Four of the participants had attended some form of LGBTQ training in the past.

The interviews were conducted in places chosen by the social workers, which in almost all cases was at their workplaces. I asked them open-ended questions about their understanding and knowledge of the needs of older trans adults as well as their knowledge of norm-critical approaches and perspectives. Norm-critical approaches aim at questioning existing societal norms as well as establishing awareness of how norms affect people's life conditions. For example, I asked what they considered to be a norm-critical approach and how they perceived their knowledge about norm-critical perspectives. The interviews lasted between 40 and 80 minutes. The social workers appeared to be interested in the topic and wanted to share their perspectives with me. They also expressed that the interviews gave them a good opportunity to reflect and identify areas to develop as well as to contribute to research. For detailed information on processing and analysing the empirical material, please see Smolle and Espvall (2021). In the results section, the social workers are assigned a number and are referred to as SW (social worker).

Profession, professionalism and room for manoeuvre

Being a social worker means being in a political field given that the municipal organisations in which social workers work are politically controlled in the sense that political perspectives and decisions play a fundamental role in shaping the legislation, guidelines and resources which inevitably affect a municipal organisation – both in terms of decision making and policy practice and discourse (Ponnert and Svensson, 2019). Because social workers are often connected to an organisation, the profession is usually described as organisation-dependent, and the organisation can therefore leave its mark on the professional role. This might imply that less space is given for continuous reflection on professionalism because the profession is so strongly connected to the guidelines and practices in organisations (Svensson, 2011; Ponnert and Svensson, 2019). It is important to mention that there is a global definition of professionalism in social work. Professionalism cannot be separated from definitions that formulate what social work is and stands for concerning social justice, human rights, diversity and collective responsibility (International Federation of Social Workers [IFSW], 2018). Meanwhile, professionalism is perhaps sometimes accredited to someone who practises according to what is expected from a person in that role from the perspective of the public as well as by upholding certain norms. Considering the latter – upholding certain norms – there is a possibility that the discourse on professionalism contains cisnormative characteristics (among other common norms), which could imply that one is considered professional if one acts according to that very norm.. It is therefore important to keep in mind that views on professionalism might vary in different contexts, such as in this study, where what the social workers mean when referring to professionalism is not always clearly defined.

To fully grasp the challenges for the professional social worker, it is of great importance to emphasise the complexity of working at the intersection of an organisation and a professional setting. However, the profession is also positioned between organisations and clients, which implies an insight into both the client's situation and the organisation's resources and rules (Lipsky, 2010 [1980]). It is here that room for manoeuvre comes into play, which can be described as a kind of choice in different settings where professionals can decide how they want to interpret and act in certain situations (Ponnert and Svensson, 2019) based on their professional knowledge and the rules that exist within the organisation as well as the client's situation. Professional competence is also necessary to successfully manage complex requirements in an ethically sound manner following, for example, the Global Social Work Statement of Ethical Principles (IFSW, 2018).

Social workers' professionalism also consists of being able to combine their profession with a professional approach, where knowledge – experiential, empirical or theoretical – is a key component for using their room for manoeuvre to find solutions for clients in complex situations. There is value in social workers working for a reflective and holistic view of the complexities in the human situation (IFSW, 2018), which is central to professionalism and is at the core of the profession (Ponnert and Svensson, 2019).

The social work perspective

The social workers interviewed in the study reflected on professionalism in various ways as well as certain challenges regarding professional setting, preparedness and how to act, as well as the methods and strategies they use. They also expressed several times that they want to do good and to support people, which is also why many chose to be social workers. Yet, they pointed out that they lack experience in supporting older trans adults and described their knowledge of trans issues as limited. Furthermore, they all spoke of the risk of offending older trans adults, for example through exclusionary language and limited knowledge, by asking questions that older adults do not understand or simply by violating privacy. Several challenges emerged from their statements in this regard. These included fears that their assumptions could result in causing offence, that scarce information about the trans experience could lead to inadequate support and that the administrative system automatically excludes people due to its inherent cisnormativity work.

The challenging setting

The setting in which the social workers practise professionally was problematised repeatedly during the interviews. It was pointed out that the settings both enable and inhibit change in various areas, such as current gender norms that are strongly perpetuated in organisations. It was particularly noticeable that the social workers described their work settings as hetero- and cisnormative:

> 'There are different expectations around men and women. If an older woman dies, a man may need help because he may have never cooked or cleaned before because it was always done by the woman in the household. We place certain expectations on what a woman and a man have to be responsible for.' (SW 15)

They also spoke about normative beliefs regarding sexuality and gender identity, where older adults are not presumed to deviate from a hetero- and cisnormative framework. Because heteronormativity and cisnormativity are deeply engrained in society, it is not very surprising that social workers, like people in general society, have learned and share those norms, even in their workplaces. Re-learning, in addition to questioning one's values and beliefs, was mentioned as being relevant but very challenging. This is due to a challenging professional setting consisting not only of individuals and their opinions but also – to a higher degree – structurally and institutionally embedded beliefs and values:

> 'It takes quite a lot to change the ideas in the workplace because if you do, you have to change everything completely as everything is structural. Even if you say that you understand and should work according to that, I think that it is so deeply rooted in many people,

and it would be difficult to change. You have grown up with these norms, for example, saying "he" and "she".' (SW 1)

Cisnormativity is deeply rooted in institutional settings and in individual professionals in our society, but without challenging the norms through, for example, norm-critical approaches, people who do not fit into the norms are made invisible. The quote thereby illustrates how cisnormativity can affect professionalism, especially when there is a lack of norm-critical or trans-affirming strategies within a professional setting.

Further, a number of organisational challenges were described concerning visibility and support of older trans adults, for instance the common use of only two pronouns when discussing older adults and colleagues or the issue rarely being prioritised in their professional settings. Both of these indicate a cisnormative practice. Therefore, it can seem like a large step for the individual social worker to adopt more trans-affirmative and norm-critical approaches when serving older trans adults, especially when this is not supported by their setting. Also, due to a lack of experiential knowledge, as none of the social workers had met an older trans adult in their professional role as far as they knew, it is likely an even bigger challenge for an individual to feel motivated to develop such approaches in their professional settings.

Social workers' concerns and preparedness for supporting older trans adults

"The risk is really that you assume a lot of things that are not true" (SW 8). This was expressed in different ways by the social workers who believed that trans people's needs to be actively prioritised in social services so that they can learn more about them and thereby provide older adults more appropriate services. There is an additional aspect to this, namely stereotypical assumptions about trans people in particular in that a person is expected to be, feel, and look a certain way simply because they are trans or have trans experiences. These assumptions also involve age norms:

> 'It's a norm that just because you're older you can't change your life choices, but even if you're 80, you might have 20 years left in your life. We can be helpful along the way, I think. But yes, this is why we need training, follow-up talks, etcetera. We need to learn how to ask questions. After that, you become comfortable doing it. Because if you are not comfortable, you might not ask those questions.' (SW 13)

The quote reveals that if the person is of a certain age and a recipient of social services, the older adult can be given professional support for better mental health in their old age and as a trans person. Yet, this seems to come with some professional concerns. One of the difficulties referred to in the quote is the challenge of asking questions in a way that makes needs visible without causing offence. The risk of offending a person, due to the incorrect use of language as a result of limited knowledge or cisnormative and/or stereotypical assumptions, was the most tangible concern as well as the most central result in the interview material:

> 'So it is important to be aware that there is a risk of offending that person. It is important that I, as an individual, fill a knowledge gap or take responsibility for my lack of knowledge about the problem. You have to be the proactive one when you are meeting the client.' (SW 7)

It is important for professionals to take responsibility for increasing their knowledge when it is lacking in an area, as is argued in the quote. This could also be seen as vital in order to fulfil ethical principles (IFSW, 2018) for social work, in other words to practise in a professional manner. In a situation like that described in the quote, there is significant room for manoeuvre in that the individual also has the opportunity to make the decision makers aware that more knowledge is needed for them to be able to adequately respond to the organisation's target group. In other words, to fulfil their responsibility and assignment: "I do not feel comfortable, and that is not good. I need more knowledge" (SW 15). Thus lack of knowledge – experiential and theoretical – leads the social worker to express professional insecurities, such as not feeling comfortable when talking about supporting older trans adults, and cisnormativity is unlikely to be challenged when knowledge is limited and strategies are not implemented, thereby affecting professional preparedness. If knowledge does not exist, and if the questions are not asked as a result of, for example, fears of causing offence, it is conceivable that potential needs are not made visible either. If that happens, it is difficult to make sure that the older adult's needs are met. To some extent, social workers who avoid asking certain questions could be seen as acting professionally in that they are actively trying to avoid offending the older adults they meet. However, this might simply result in not asking important questions. Meanwhile, some of the respondents expressed that they were unsure about which needs older trans adults might have in contrast to cisgender people. One explained:

> 'You need to know the conditions these people have lived under and how these can conceivably affect their needs. I can't comment on that, but I assume that they have lived hidden or with a forced gender. Of course, it affects them if they have lived like this all their lives. But I don't know how.' (SW 14)

There was some understanding that past experiences, such as living in hiding, can affect older trans adults' current needs. For example, some might need support in 'coming out' as older adults or need support with experiencing thoughts and feelings associated with gender dysphoria. The quote also illustrates the need for professionals to know more about this in order to feel better prepared to meet the needs of older trans adults: "There is some insecurity that even if you have some theoretical knowledge, that won't really help when meeting a person" (SW 7). The social workers in this study had some sort of experiential knowledge that makes them professionally prepared for future meetings with any clients; however, they seemed to feel insecure about a lack of experience from not previously meeting older trans adults. It is questioned by the social workers if theoretical knowledge would be enough for feeling professionally prepared for supporting this specific group of older adults. Knowledge might, however, not be enough for everyone and every situation, and thus methods and strategies for preparedness and adequate support should be further explored.

Work methods and strategies

Work methods and strategies that were generally described as helpful in the social workers' work were also said to be problematic or challenging due to their hetero- and cisnormative design. Several social workers talked about the practical strategies they use to ask questions, for instance a standard questionnaire that contains predetermined themes with associated questions. This covers everything from cooking and the household to hygiene and is meant to be relatively comprehensive for how the person lives, what they can manage on their own, what they need help with and what their wishes for support are. However, several social workers pointed out that they do not follow the guide because they know roughly what questions to ask. Several also stated that nothing in the questionnaire led to any questions being asked about needs relating to trans identity or trans experience. Furthermore, it emerged that work methods for responding to older trans adults were not named anywhere, and the only thing that appears is that everyone must be treated equally: "I don't think it is addressed in the documents [official documents for/in the organisation]. It probably doesn't address anything about gender identity, other than the fact that we should treat everyone equally" (SW 14). Equal treatment was repeatedly mentioned during the interviews. This is also at the core of the profession itself and appears in guidelines, ethical codes (IFSW, 2018) and national legislation (Swedish Discrimination Act 2008; Ponnert and Svensson, 2019). The respondents said that even though cisnormativity is evident in the work, and knowledge about older trans adults is limited among social workers, the important thing is that everyone is treated in the same way by professionals in the social services. When they were asked to give examples or describe what it means to treat everyone equally in practice, there was not a uniform answer, and some had difficulties in responding. What the respondents seemed to be aiming for (and seemed to be referring to) is that everyone should be treated with respect and given the same opportunities for services, rather than that everyone should be given the same support or services no matter what (Fineman, 2010; Anderson et al, 2018; RFSL and Siverskog, 2021; Smolle and Espvall, 2021; Smolle and Siverskog, 2023). To do so, knowledge about and understanding of groups and how they are affected by societal structures and cisnormativity and how they are treated by people in society is essential. Another social worker continued on the same theme of equal treatment:

> 'We sometimes talk about the fact that we are an authority and that everyone should be treated equally, but then, how it works in practice ... So we can talk about gender, that a person should not be disadvantaged because of it when they apply for assistance. The norms should not matter, for example, regarding what a person is expected to do based on one's gender, but it is more of a loose discussion. Nothing is written down, and it is perhaps more something that we talk about casually sometimes.' (SW 15)

Because the perspective of equal treatment appears in the IFSW ethical principles as well as in Swedish legislation (Discrimination Act 2008), there is some form of foundation for practice. Nevertheless, as mentioned previously, the social workers interviewed for this study lack experience in supporting older trans adults, which means they lack clarity about how to proceed in the practical application of guidelines and legislation. However, based on the previous quote, as well as several of the quotes in this chapter, the social workers show that they have thought about the issues to some extent but have not managed to implement strategies or working methods that could be described as norm-critical or trans-affirmative.

The administrative systems social workers use currently feature only two gender options. There are currently only two gender options, and there is a box that is usually filled in based on the personal identity number (gendered in Sweden). This means that social workers have an idea in advance of who (in other words, which gender) is applying for care interventions, regardless of how the person identifies. Non-binary people are made invisible and are even excluded by the wording. Furthermore, the systems do not recognise other experiences of gender identity and gender expression even in more binary forms, for example the experience of varying between gender categories. Consequently, the validity of the answers decreases when the questions and answers do not reflect the person's perceived reality.

The social workers also referred to the challenge of asking questions in ways that differ from what they are used to, perhaps based on a norm-critical approach, which should be expected from the authorities (in their words). One social worker described what needs to be improved in this area:

> 'To depart from all the old norms that we still have. To ask questions that are outside the framework that we have today. ... To put absolutely no value on something that is probably very common for people to do. Not only having "Male" and "Female" to choose from. To ask, "Which pronoun do you want me to use for you in the documents?" for example. It's only one question. We don't ask that today, because we take it for granted that it's a male or female when we meet the person. It's stupid. But if you look into that field a little, some may be offended if you go deeper. That is difficult.' (SW 10)

The quote illustrates the worry of offending people through the use of language and work methods. Specifically, this social worker mentions having options other than 'male' and 'female' in forms and questionnaires and also states that it would be good to ask people about their pronouns to open up to variation and avoid assuming gender and pronouns. However, they said that this is not something that they currently do, and this is largely due to the risk of causing offence. Another social worker (15) adds another reason for not asking about pronouns:

> 'I haven't asked what pronoun a person wants to be addressed with, I think it feels awkward for me. But it could be a good way to do it. I don't know how I could make it happen though. Another way is to just mention a person by name, so you don't have to think about pronouns, but then I think that the documents become very difficult to read, only name name name name.' (SW 15)

A certain level of resistance is also indicated in this quote, but unlike the previous quote about the risk of causing offence, this respondent highlights the potential of feeling uncomfortable in situations with older adults as a professional. However, asking for pronouns is suggested as a good work method in this quote too.

What can we learn from this?

As far as they were aware, the social workers participating in this study had never met older trans adults in a professional context. It is likely that even if the social workers had met this group, it would not be acknowledged because of the general assumption about older adults being cisgender (Siverskog,

2016; SOU, 2017) as well as the lack of strategies for making this group more visible to social services (Smolle and Espvall, 2021). Yet they have nevertheless thought about trans issues and built up a certain preparedness, although this seems to be affected by discourses on professionalism where offending is the main concern instead of how to achieve trans-affirmative services. The concerns therefore seem to stand in the way of, or even counteract, professional preparedness, because they avoid acknowledging trans issues due to insecurities. For example, they expressed worries about the risk of causing offence when asking about pronouns, and because of these insecurities, they avoid asking these questions. This reinforces cisnormativity within social services. Asking about pronouns may seem like a trivial issue and potentially less of a challenge. However, asking about pronouns could help to open further conversations, and social workers might miss out on something that could be important to the person they meet. This could be one strategy to challenge cisnormativity in their professional settings.

The social workers interviewed in this study want to do right by the older adults they meet but contribute to making the needs of older trans adults invisible. This calls for the implementation of norm-critical approaches to challenge both what is considered professional (through discourses) and to be able to support older adults according to Swedish legislation and according to ethical principles (IFSW, 2018). Professional preparedness would also likely be strengthened by the implementation of such approaches.

As mentioned earlier, there are ambitions at several levels to strengthen protection for trans people in society. For this to be possible, organisations that provide support to trans people in need of care must provide adequate services. At the same time, we are not yet there. Many previous studies indicate that older trans people experience concerns about negative treatment and a lack of understanding and knowledge among the professionals who are supposed to provide help (Siverskog, 2014; Löf and Olaison, 2018). Simultaneously, this study indicates that social workers who meet older adults and determine service needs lack experience in supporting trans people as well as knowledge about trans-related issues. Trans people's needs are invisible in organisations where the social workers' practice and trans-related issues are not a priority. It is therefore not particularly surprising that social workers' knowledge of trans people's needs is limited and cisnormativity is not challenged. It is thus evident that social workers, or others who meet older adults in need of support and help, need more trans-affirmative knowledge (theoretical and experiential) to make trans issues as well as the potential needs of older trans adults visible in social services. It is thus conceivable that social workers would experience fewer insecurities and be more prepared to support older trans adults in their professional practice, and older trans adults can thus hopefully experience greater confidence (concerning receiving adequate services) when in need of care and support from social services.

Because social workers practise in complex situations where they need to relate not only to the client but also to the organisation's regulations, there are rarely simple solutions, and this makes decision making difficult at times (Lipsky, 2010 [1980]). Further, in today's society, organisations, as well as the profession, are characterised by a market logic, which affects how resources and interests are assessed. This largely influences which issues are prioritised within the organisations (Ponnert and Svensson, 2019). What is evident in this study is that issues regarding gender identity and gender expression are not prioritised within municipal social services. This should be considered a problem given the reports on transgender health (for example SOU, 2017, p 92) and the need for adequate support. Social workers have a responsibility to highlight these issues by using their experiential and theoretical knowledge and room for manoeuvre, as well as providing safe spaces for older trans adults by adapting norm-critical approaches and self-reflexivity. However, the issues need to be prioritised at a higher level (politically and organisationally) so that social workers have appropriate guidelines from which to work and reasonable resources are allocated. This, together with the strategies, could help social workers experience more professional preparedness to act ethically (IFSW, 2018), to challenge cisnormativity and to provide trans-affirmative care and support.

References

Anderson, A.R., Knee, E., Ramos, W.D. and Quash, T.M. (2018) '"We just treat everyone the same": LGBTQ aquatic management strategies, barriers and implementation', *International Journal of Aquatic Research and Education*, 11(1): article 2.

Bremer, S. (2011) 'Kroppslinjer: kön, transsexualism och kropp i berättelser om könskorrigering' [Bodylines: gender, transsexualism and embodiment in narratives on gender correction], PhD thesis, University of Gothenburg.

European Commission (2020) 'Union of equality: LGBTIQ equality strategy 2020–2025'.

Fineman, M.A. (2010) 'The vulnerable subject and the responsive state', *Emory Law Journal*, 60(2): 251–75.

Fredriksen-Goldsen, K.I., Kim, H.-J., Barkan, S.E., Muraco, A. and Hoy-Ellis, C.P. (2013) 'Health disparities among lesbian, gay, and bisexual older adults: results from a population-based study', *American Journal of Public Health*, 103(10): 1802–9, Available from: https://doi.org/10.2105/AJPH.2012.301110

Grant, J.M., Mottet, L., Tanis, J.E., Harrison, J., Herman, J. and Keisling, M. (2011) 'Injustice at every turn: a report of the national transgender discrimination survey', Washington: National Center for Transgender Equality.

International Federation of Social Workers (IFSW) (2018) 'Global social work statement of ethical principles', Available from: https://www.ifsw.org/global-social-work-statement-of-ethical-principles/

Kattari, S.K., Kinney, K., Kattari, L. and Walls, E. (2020) 'Introduction to social work and health care with transgender and nonbinary individuals and communities', in S.K. Kattari, K. Kinney, L. Kattari and E. Walls (eds) *Social Work and Health Care Practice with Transgender and Nonbinary Individuals and Communities*, Abingdon: Taylor & Francis, pp 1–10.

Linander, I., Alm, E., Goicolea, I. and Harryson, L. (2019) '"It was like I had to fit into a category": care-seekers' experiences of gender regulation in the Swedish trans-specific healthcare', *Health*, 23(1): 21–38, Available from: https://doi.org/10.1177/1363459317708824

Lipsky, M. (2010 [1980]) *Street-Level Bureaucracy: Dilemmas of the Individual in Public Services*, New York: Russell Sage Foundation.

Löf, J. and Olaison, A. (2018) '"I don't want to go back into the closet just because I need care": recognition of older LGBTQ adults in relation to future care needs', *European Journal of Social Work*, 23(2): 253–64.

Ponnert, L. and Svensson, K. (2019) *Socionomen i myndigheten: att göra gott, göra rätt och göra nytta* [The social worker in the public authority: To do good, do right and be useful], Malmö: Gleerups Utbildning AB.

Public Health Agency of Sweden (Folkhälsomyndigheten) (2015) 'Hälsan och hälsans bestämningsfaktorer för transpersoner: en rapport om hälsoläget bland transpersoner i Sverige' [Health and the determinants of health for transgender people: a report on the health situation among trans people in Sweden], Folkhälsomyndigheten.

Siverskog, A. (2014) '"They just don't have a clue": transgender aging and implications for social work', *Journal of Gerontological Social Work*, 57(2–4): 386–406, Available from: https://doi.org/10.1080/01634372.2014.895472

Siverskog, A. (2016) 'Queera livslopp: att leva och åldras som LHBTQ-person i en heteronormativ värld' [Queer life courses: to live and grow old as a LGBTQ person in a heteronormative world], PhD thesis, Linköping University, Linkoping University Electronic Press, Available from: https://doi.org/10.3384/diss.diva-132553

Smolle, S. and Espvall, M. (2021) 'Transgender competence in social work with older adults', *Journal of Social Service Research*, 47(4): 522–36, Available from: https://doi.org/10.1080/01488376.2020.1848968

Smolle, S. and Siverskog, A. (2023) 'Transgender, human rights and social work', in S. Webb (ed) *The Routledge Handbook of Critical Social Work*, Abingdon: Routledge, pp 586–98.

SOU (2017:92) Transpersoner i Sverige: förslag till stärkt ställning och bättre levnadsvillkor; betänkande av utredningen om stärkt ställning och bättre levnadsvillkor för transpersoner' [Transgender people in Sweden: suggestions for a stronger position and better living conditions; report of the investigations on strengthened position and better living conditions for transgender people], Regeringskansliet.

Summanen, E. (2023) 'Trans och kön: en introduktion' [Trans and gender: an introduction], in E. Summanen and M. Wurm (eds) *Trans: fakta, forskning och erfarenheter* [Trans: facts, research and experiences], Stockholm: Natur & Kultur, pp 15–35.

Svensson, L.G. (2011) 'Profession, organisation, kollegialitet och ansvar' [Profession, organisation, collegiality and responsibility], *Socialvetenskaplig tidskrift*, 18(4): 301–19.

Swedish Federation for Lesbian, Gay, Bisexual, Transgender, Queer and Intersex Rights (RFSL) and Siverskog, A. (2021) 'Queer äldreomsorg? Att möta äldre lhbtq-personer inom vård och omsorg' [Queer elderly care? Meeting older LGBTQ people in health and social care settings], RFSL Stockholm.

Vincent, G.K. and Velkoff, V.A. (2010) 'The next four decades: the older population in the United States; 2010 to 2050', Washington: US Census Bureau.

8

Gender-affirming surgery in later life: centring older adults' perspectives to promote equitable access and person-centred surgical care

Elijah R. Castle and Laura L. Kimberly

Introduction

Gender-affirming surgery in older adults is an often-overlooked aspect of healthcare for transgender and gender diverse (TGD) populations (Gamble et al, 2020). Older adults may not be perceived as appropriate surgical candidates based on age-related assumptions about patient preferences and postoperative outcomes. Moreover, older age may intersect with race/ ethnicity and gender identity to compound inequities in access to quality care for older TGD individuals, particularly for older TGD persons of colour (Bloemen et al, 2019; Javier, 2019). Access to financial resources (Javier, 2019); health education, especially as information in the TGD community is more widely shared in online spaces (Cipolletta et al, 2017); and lack of information specific to gender-affirming surgery and sexuality (Javier, 2019) for older TGD individuals can present further barriers. To date, older TGD-identifying adults' perspectives have remained largely absent from the discourse on gender-affirming surgery, including desire for surgery, access to surgical procedures and postoperative needs and support.

This chapter examines theoretical and practical considerations for older TGD individuals who have undergone or may desire gender-affirming surgery. The authors are based in New York City, United States. Thus, while we have made sure to include data and perspectives from beyond our geographic location, our frame of reference is informed by gender-affirming surgery and trans populations within the US, especially as it pertains to insurance and public policy. One of us is transgender and one of us is cisgender, and we both have professional experience in gender-affirming surgery research within a large academic medical centre. Our approach to this work is framed by our lived personal and professional experience in transgender medicine and surgery, bioethics, gerontological social work and social policy, and surgical practice more broadly. We focus on the importance of amplifying older adults' perspectives to inform patient-centred care and underscore the need for strong community and social support to ultimately ensure respectful and competent care for older TGD individuals.

While of course there are trans people of all ages who do not seek gender-affirming medical interventions, the focus of this chapter is on gender-affirming surgery and the barriers and other considerations that may factor into older trans adults' healthcare experiences. To begin, we will address how older age may impact pathways to gender-affirming surgery, including how ageism factors into access to care and surgical decision making, as well as how a lack of long-term outcomes data for gender-affirming surgery (Agochukwu-Mmonu et al, 2021) impacts older individuals navigating postoperative healthcare needs as they age. This discussion will explore how insufficient trans competency in various care-based settings (Bloemen et al, 2019; Javier, 2019) can impede access to surgery and compromise postoperative care. Lastly, we consider the role of social support for older TGD individuals (Javier, 2019; Gamble et al, 2020; Pereira and Banerjee, 2021) and strategies for supporting this population as they undergo gender-affirming surgery.

Gendered embodiment and ageism

Gendered embodiment

In this chapter, we use the term embodiment to refer to the 'experience of living in, perceiving, and experiencing the world from the physical and material places of our bodies' (DeLamater and Plante, 2015). The reasons trans people opt for medical transition vary. Generally speaking, medical transition is typically sought for the purpose of aligning one's physical body with one's ideal or authentic sense of gendered embodiment (Kennis et al, 2022). This may include altering primary or secondary sex characteristics to become more typical conceptions of male or female phenotypes, to be able to more easily wear clothes that are aligned with their gender and to improve sexual wellbeing (Kennis et al, 2022). Gender-affirming medical interventions can help achieve these goals (Robinson et al, 2021; Kennis et al, 2022; Kloer et al, 2023). Gendered embodiment can therefore be positively framed as an achievement of a desired physicality and way of moving through the world. However, stereotypes of gendered embodiment, such as men being strong and women being fragile (DeLamater and Plante, 2015), can contribute to the surveillance and criticism of those whose bodies do not conform to gendered norms, including the bodies of trans people.

Intersection of ageism with other forms of stigma

Older adults experience the effects of normative ideas of gendered embodiment as well. For example, the idea of the 'little old lady' evokes the image of a small, weak woman and connotes fragility (Grenier and Hanley, 2007). This stereotype can lead people and institutions to interact with and perceive older women in ways that may not reflect their own perceptions of self or how they live their lives (Grenier and Hanley, 2007). The World Health Organization (WHO) defines ageism as the ways in which we stereotype and discriminate against people based on age (WHO, 2021). The term originated in 1969 with Robert Butler specifically in reference to older adults, though his definition is expansive and includes younger individuals as well (Butler, 1969; Achenbaum, 2015). Importantly, Butler's definition also acknowledges the intersection of age with race and class and how these compound oppression, discrimination and societal disenfranchisement (Butler, 1969).

Ageism interacts with sexuality as well. Often, literature on sexuality in later life cites the fact that older adults are not perceived as sexual beings, which may affect their lived experiences and the care they receive (Towler et al, 2021). For example, older adults more frequently broach the topic of sexual health and sexuality, as compared with their providers (Agochukwu-Mmonu et al, 2021). Yet, older adults may desire to maintain their sexuality and capacity to have sex through medical interventions (DeLamater and Plante, 2015). This could include taking medications to improve erectile quality or treat vaginal atrophy or having an erectile device surgically implanted (Holzapfel, 1994; Rosen, 1996; DeLamater and Plante, 2015). Recognising the sexual health needs and sexuality of older adults can help prevent the need for their continual self-advocacy in clinical settings and beyond and create opportunities for more resources and education for this group, particularly for older trans adults.

Given the impact of multiply marginalised identities on lived experience (Crenshaw, 1989), being trans *and* older may result in experiencing compounded stigma (Waling et al, 2020). Even with improved access to healthcare and gender-affirming medical interventions and increased societal acceptance in some contexts, trans individuals face stigma on many levels. Stigmatised groups and individuals within those groups face limited access to resources, social isolation and stress (Hatzenbuehler et al, 2013). For example, as a result of structural stigma, trans individuals often have difficulty finding clinicians who are equipped to treat them with competence (Poteat et al, 2013; McCrone, 2018). Other examples of systemic and structural stigma for trans individuals include a lack of institutions built to support trans people, such as shelters or treatment centres (Poteat et al, 2013). Stigma may affect in which spaces trans individuals feel safe, and trans individuals may limit opportunities they have in order to avoid continued experiences of being stigmatised (Poteat et al, 2013). Overall, trans individuals report negative experiences with clinicians, and clinicians report being uncomfortable or not knowing how to provide competent care to trans individuals (Poteat et al, 2013). While much has been published on gender-affirming healthcare and surgery, clinicians often lack specific training in gender-affirming medical care (Klein and Golub, 2020) and instead must extrapolate from knowledge that is similar to what is necessary for transgender healthcare but lacks data specific to this demographic. Klein and Golub (2020), for instance, highlight the lack of information about trans masculine patients' experiences of and preferences for conversations specific to sexual health and anatomy, and the lack of assessment tools for engaging in these conversations.

Trans individuals often have difficulty finding competent clinicians who can provide gender-affirming care (Puckett et al, 2018), as well as clinicians with whom and environments in which they feel safe (Fredriksen-Goldsen et al, 2014). Some individuals opt to travel for high-quality care (Puckett et al, 2018), but this is not a feasible option for those who do not have the resources, mobility or energy to go elsewhere. Further, identifying a clinician willing to provide care does not necessarily mean that the clinician or other staff will be competent. Generally speaking, older adults tend to have more trouble finding competent providers whom they trust (Goins et al, 2005). Bias and stigma in medical environments are also widespread and longstanding problems for trans people, and the severity of this can range from feeling uncomfortable in a medical setting to experiencing abuse and explicit harassment (Puckett et al, 2018). It is important to take into account how these experiences are layered and relevant across care delivery contexts, highlighting the relevance of community support.

Gender-affirming surgery in older age

Published research reveals the dearth of data on outcomes of gender-affirming surgery in older adults. Studies typically include patient populations with an average age of between 30 and 39 (De Cuypere et al, 2005; Monstrey et al, 2008; Rossi Neto et al, 2012; Amend et al, 2013; Buncamper et al, 2016; Acar et al, 2022; Blickensderfer et al, 2023). While a few studies report on patients into their 70s (Massie et al, 2018; Boas et al, 2019), most have a maximum age in the 50 to 59 range (Blanchard et al, 1987; Berry et al, 2012; Donato et al, 2017; Wolf and Kwartin, 2021) with a follow-up period of three years or less (Goddard et al, 2007; Frederick et al, 2017; Gaither et al, 2018; Timmermans et al, 2023). Mastectomy and vaginoplasty/vulvoplasty tend to be most commonly addressed (Massie et al, 2018; Boas et al, 2019; Pittelkow et al, 2020; Acar et al, 2022; Skorochod et al, 2023). The association between age and surgical outcomes presents an important consideration in the context of gender-affirming surgery for older patients. While many older people fare well following surgical procedures, older adults generally are seen as higher-risk surgical patients (Finlayson and Birkmeyer, 2001; Watt et al, 2018). And although chronological age can be an indicator of increased likelihood of poor surgical outcomes (Finlayson and Birkmeyer,

2001), oftentimes it serves as a proxy for factors such as frailty status and other comorbidities which offer a more accurate estimate of surgical risk (Xue, 2011; Shih et al, 2015; Townsend and Robinson, 2015; Watt et al, 2018). In particular, frailty is a clinically recognised vulnerability which is associated with ageing (Xue, 2011). A variety of instruments have been developed to measure frailty and commonly include low grip strength, low energy, slow walking speed/gait, low physical activity, weight loss, delirium, recent falls and urinary incontinence (Xue, 2011). A review of National Surgical Quality Improvement Program (NSQIP)[1] data specific to plastic surgery indicated that age itself is a risk factor only for individuals 80 years of age and older (Shih et al, 2015), with a similar conclusion reached regarding free flap reconstructive surgeries (Sorg et al, 2023). For patients undergoing urologic care, the Charlson comorbidity index can help assess for risk preoperatively (Townsend and Robinson, 2015). Wounds also tend to have a longer healing time in older adults, presenting the potential for further postoperative complications (Wicke et al, 2009). While age appears to be a factor, wound healing can also be affected by cigarette smoking/nicotine use, diabetes, peripheral artery disease and chronic venous insufficiency (Wicke et al, 2009).

Older adults may need more support than younger patients when recovering from surgery and healing wounds, and a preoperative frailty assessment can help inform what may be needed relative to postoperative support. As an increasing number of older adults undergo surgery, the use of a multidisciplinary collaborative care team can enhance recovery in surgical contexts (Kehlet, 1997). The *enhanced recovery after surgery*, or ERAS, protocol was developed to address the following factors to improve surgical recovery: preoperative education, enteral nutrition, reduced stress, pain relief, exercise/ambulation and growth factors (Kehlet, 1997). Surgical outcomes data from colorectal cancer surgery (Martínez-Escribano et al, 2022), lumber fusion surgery (Cui et al, 2022) and knee arthroplasty procedures (Li et al, 2023) in older adults indicate that following an ERAS protocol can improve surgical outcomes, as compared to outcomes in patients whose treatment is not guided by an ERAS protocol. Evidence for the use of ERAS protocols in surgical care also emphasises the importance of a multidisciplinary, collaborative approach which focuses not only on a successful surgery but on attentive, robust pre- and postoperative care as well. These considerations suggest that a patient-centred and individualised approach to gender-affirming surgical care for older people can confer meaningful benefit.

What assistive technologies specific to postoperative genitals might benefit older trans adults?

Some individuals may have problems implementing integral aspects of postoperative care for some gender-affirming surgeries. Thus, it is important to consider how assistive technologies may help resolve such problems. One example is vaginal dilation, which individuals who undergo vaginoplasty must perform for the remainder of their lives to prevent the canal from closing as a result of scar tissue. Dilation must be performed on a regular basis. Initially it is very often, and as time goes on, dilation can be performed weekly or even less often. For most individuals, though, dilation must remain a regular part of their routine genital care. Dilation generally requires an individual to be able to reach their genitals, and the flexibility and strength in one's arms and wrists to manipulate the dilator into one's body at the right angle, hold it there, and then remove it. They must also be able to apply the lubricant to the dilator, and then clean the canal and the rest of their genitals afterward. This would be a difficult task for anyone with limited mobility or vision and is a concern for anyone who is disabled or experiencing cognitive impairment, which includes many older adults, especially those at the later end of the age spectrum. To help individuals maintain their bodily integrity as they age, it is important to find feasible solutions for these issues.

Ageing after surgery

For those who are *ageing after surgery*, we refer to trans individuals who undergo gender-affirming surgery earlier in life and then transition into older age. Much of the gender-affirming surgery literature reports short-term postoperative outcomes, typically one or two years. Most of the surgical literature reports on trans individuals who are between the ages of 30 and 39, and there are, on average, only a few years of follow-up at most. Long-term outcomes data reporting how individuals fare as they age into their 50s, 60s, 70s and beyond are essentially nonexistent. The lack of data also reflects trends in support for gender-affirming medical interventions through the last century. Trans people have sought out gender-affirming medical care for decades: the first recorded gender-affirming surgery took place in 1931 (Meyerowitz, 2009; Stryker, 2009). Yet institutions providing this care have frequently been forced to shutter their programmes due to political or other ideological opposition to trans care (Denny, 2002; Shuster, 2021). As a result, long-term follow-up data on gender-affirming surgeries are not widely available, and ongoing attempts to curtail or prohibit institutions from providing medical care to trans people continue to present roadblocks.

How does surgically (re)constructed anatomy fare through the ageing process?

Very little data exist regarding how surgically reconstructed genitals age for trans populations. This is true as well for other kinds of genital reconstruction surgeries performed on individuals at younger ages (Wang and Poppas,

2017) and is due in part to the difficulty of gathering long-term follow-up data (Goddard et al, 2007). Thus little is known about how surgically reconstructed genitals may change through the ageing process, or what kind of long-term follow up care may be needed. For example, some cisgender women undergoing menopause may benefit from supplementation with exogenous hormones in order to prevent or treat vaginal atrophy. Whether this is the case for transgender women and trans feminine individuals who underwent vaginoplasty in their 20s or 30s is unknown.

Additionally, trans individuals who undergo phalloplasty may have an erectile device implanted, yet there is a lack of data regarding how these devices fare long term (Boskey et al, 2022; Purohit et al, 2022). Information provided to patients is often based on data from cisgender men who undergo erectile device implantation (Preto et al, 2020). However, little is known about how long these implants may last for trans individuals and whether there may be a need for replacement at an older age. It is also unclear whether individuals who undergo phalloplasty may experience any changes or thinning in the skin of their penis or scrotum, which may increase the risk of erosion of an erectile device or testicular implants. These questions are not intended to incite concern but rather to emphasise the need for long-term follow-up data to better inform ongoing care and support for older surgical patients.

Gender-affirming surgery and long-term care

Beyond provision of medical care in healthcare settings, concerns about trans-competent care are perhaps even more pronounced in institutional long-term care settings. Many adults aged 65 and over will need long-term care at some point as they age (Kaye et al, 2010). Few studies describe the experiences of older adults in nursing homes (Greenwood et al, 2018), which impose restrictions on independence and autonomy that are enforced by the policies and structure of the institutional context. The lack of autonomy and control over one's physical body and environment can compound feelings of isolation and emphasise a general feeling of decline in one's quality of life (Towler et al, 2021). In addition to these institutional constraints on autonomy, there are also the physical restrictions resulting from bodily changes that come with ageing and a lack of societal and technological infrastructure to mitigate these physical limitations in order to maintain social integration and positive quality of life for older and disabled individuals (Davis, 2016).

Access to long-term care is a concern for many trans individuals as they grow older (Pang et al, 2019), and there are limited resources to support older trans adults (Catlett et al, 2023). Moreover, trans individuals often do not have many options for long-term care. Quality of care in long-term care facilities is highly variable, and numerous health and safety risks have drawn widespread criticism (Waling et al, 2020). Staff in care facilities commonly assume that residents are straight and cisgender (Bauer et al, 2013), impacting provision of appropriate care and support for their healthcare needs including long-term postsurgical care. Needs that fall beyond the range of those anticipated in cisgender individuals may go unnoticed. Even when acknowledged, competence in attending to trans-specific needs may be limited or nonexistent. Interviews with older trans adults reflect these concerns. For example, in a study by Pang et al, one participant reflected that bodily differences can lead to 'othering', even in environments that claim to be trans friendly (Pang et al, 2019). Participants also reported fear around loss of dignity and autonomy when living in a discriminatory facility (Pang et al, 2019). One participant went as far as to state a desire for euthanasia over long-term care (Pang et al, 2019). Unsurprisingly, given the deficits in long-term care for older trans adults, trans individuals often turn to their community for care in later life rather than relying on formal institutions (Shiu et al, 2016; Waling et al, 2022).

Community support

Community and peer support are often hugely influential in the lives of trans individuals. Despite the impact of family rejection (George et al, 2015; Chang et al, 2018) and lack of support that older trans adults may have from clinicians or other institutions and formal support systems, informal social support found through membership in a community with other trans individuals offers another key resource that has not been fully explored in these conversations (Harner, 2021). Trans individuals do often have robust intracommunity support (Harner, 2021). Social support can be protective and lead to a higher quality of life (Fredriksen-Goldsen et al, 2014; George et al, 2015; Chang et al, 2018; Castle et al, 2022). Especially when pursuing surgery, trans individuals find social and peer support to be helpful above and beyond other kinds of support (Castle et al, 2022). Often, trans individuals find support through groups (Cipolletta et al, 2017). These groups can be both in-person and online but are often easier to access online due to limitations resulting from geographic location, lack of mobility and so on. However, online options may put older adults at a disadvantage if they feel less comfortable accessing online methods of support due to lower levels of digital literacy (Hargittai et al, 2019). This can be compounded by financial inequity, both with regard to skill level and overall access (Hargittai et al, 2019).

Despite potential concerns about online access, intracommunity support is an important resource for many community members, and especially for older adults (Catlett et al, 2023), who often need more support with activities of daily living. As is evident from many examples throughout the AIDS crisis, LGBTQ+ community members have often had to care for one another because they were otherwise neglected by greater society (McCann, 1990). Intracommunity support can allow for creative approaches and solutions for providing care outside of long-term care settings. For example, the idea of communal or cooperative living as an alternative to institutionalised long-term care may be appealing to some (Waling et al, 2020). Another unconventional approach to long-term care is the use of healthcare advocates who are not family members (Catlett et al, 2023), which is especially important to identify as a possibility for those who are no longer in touch with or close to their families of origin. Finally, researchers and clinicians continue to share knowledge of best practices for transgender healthcare, but given the field's rapid evolution, social networks also play an important role in disseminating information, particularly within the trans community, where knowledge is often shared via word of mouth.

Conclusion and a call to action

Much of the discussion in this chapter centres on concerns about the current state of healthcare for older trans adults. While these concerns may be well founded, they also underscore opportunities for improvements in education, training, care delivery and research. These suggestions are summarised in Figure 8.1.

Potential solutions to the lack of healthcare resources include widening access through telehealth services, though older adults may need support with online platforms or may have trouble accessing them (Catlett et al, 2023). Education for clinicians and staff in long-term care facilities could also serve to improve the experiences for older trans adults, as well as provide them with higher-quality healthcare. Better experiences accessing healthcare will lead to individuals feeling more willing to seek out healthcare services and clinicians. Those working with older adults should strive to avoid stereotyping or making assumptions. As noted earlier, clinicians often assume their patients are cisgender and heterosexual; clinicians should be encouraged to ask about individual's gender identities and sexual orientations when relevant, to ensure their healthcare is individualised and tailored to their specific healthcare needs. Second, if a clinician learns their patient is trans, this may lead to assumptions about their healthcare or surgical desires, their bodies and anatomy and their HIV status or presence of sexually transmitted infections. Approaching patients with an open mind and asking questions to ascertain their needs for their healthcare can help to align care provision with a patient's values and goals. Multidisciplinary care is important as well for those with health conditions that need to be managed alongside their surgical care, as well as to ensure support for mental health and other needs.

Figure 8.1: Recommendations to improve the state of gender-affirming surgical care for older trans adults

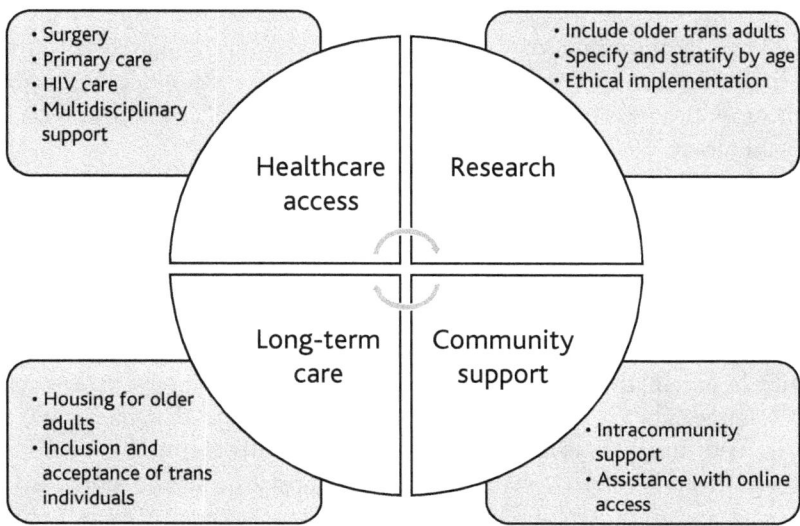

It is clear from the literature reviewed in this chapter that more data on surgical outcomes are needed to better guide patient-centred decision making and provision of gender-affirming surgery to older patients. Future research should include older trans adults, and stratifying analyses by research participant age may help to contextualise research findings and elucidate age-related trends. This is especially important in surgical outcomes reporting, where older trans adults are often not included. Surgical outcomes data can be of value in stratifying complications and by age and assessing predictive factors to enable clinicians and patients to set realistic expectations for preoperative course and anticipated postoperative recovery. Longer-term follow up with surgical patients will also strengthen the evidence base for long-term surgical outcomes to further inform evaluation for surgical candidacy, surgical care and long-term primary and sexual healthcare for patients who have undergone gender-affirming surgery. It is of utmost importance that research efforts be undertaken ethically and in partnership with trans communities. Trans individuals should be involved in all aspects of the research process, from study design to implementation and dissemination of research findings. First and foremost, research should be intended to benefit the community (Klein and Golub, 2022a, 2022b).

Aside from healthcare, other long-term care needs include stable and inclusive housing and long-term care facilities, such as rehabilitation centres and nursing homes, which can respect and competently provide care for their trans residents. Long-term care facilities as well as clinicians can help foster community support for trans individuals by referring to support groups, LGBTQ+ community centres and other community-based resources. For instance, community centres can help to provide older trans adults with support accessing online resources, when needed, for those with less digital literacy.

Much of the medically and surgically oriented scholarship on aging tends to focus on the negative aspects of aging: physical decline and disability, lack of family support, lack of competent and available healthcare resources, and more. A more positive reframing can focus on the life-enhancing aspects of gender-affirming care for older trans adults. Access to gender-affirming surgery for older trans adults may enable them to feel fully embodied and finally living in their desired embodiment. For those who had surgery at a younger age, it can feel joyous to age in a body that feels right for them. And finally, finding support with other trans community members can significantly improve social cohesion, provide needed psychosocial resources and mitigate some of the more negative aspects of trans people's healthcare experiences.

Note

[1] NSQIP is the American College of Surgeons (ACS) National Surgical Quality Improvement Program (NSQIP), a US-based verification programme for surgical quality improvement (ACS NSQIP, nd).

References

Acar, O., Alcantar, J., Millman, A., Naha, U., Cedeno, J.D., Morgantini, L. et al (2022) 'Outcomes of penile inversion vaginoplasty and robotic-assisted peritoneal flap vaginoplasty in obese and nonobese patients', *Neurourology and Urodynamics*, 42(5): 939–46. DOI: 10.1002/nau.25077

Achenbaum, W.A. (2015) 'A history of ageism since 1969', *Generations*, 39(3): 10–16, Available from: https://www.ingentaconnect.com/content/asag/gen/2015/00000039/00000003/art00003

ACS NSQIP (nd) 'ACS', Available from: https://www.facs.org/quality-programs/data-and-registries/acs-nsqip/

Agochukwu-Mmonu, N., Malani, P.N., Wittmann, D., Kirch, M., Kullgren, J., Singer, D. et al (2021) 'Interest in sex and conversations about sexual health with health care providers among older U.S. adults', *Clinical Gerontologist*, 44(3): 299–306. DOI: 10.1080/07317115.2021.1882637

Amend, B., Seibold, J., Toomey, P., Stenzl, A. and Sievert, K.-D. (2013) 'Surgical reconstruction for male-to-female sex reassignment', *European Urology*, 64(1): 141–9. DOI: 10.1016/j.eururo.2012.12.030

Bauer, M., McAuliffe, L., Nay, R. and Chenco, C. (2013) 'Sexuality in older adults: effect of an education intervention on attitudes and beliefs of residential aged care staff', *Educational Gerontology*, 39(2): 82–91. DOI: 10.1080/03601277.2012.682953

Berry, M.G., Curtis, R. and Davies, D. (2012) 'Female-to-male transgender chest reconstruction: a large consecutive, single-surgeon experience', *Journal of Plastic, Reconstructive & Aesthetic Surgery: JPRAS*, 65(6): 711–19. DOI: 10.1016/j.bjps.2011.11.053

Blanchard, R., Legault, S. and Lindsay, W.R. (1987) 'Vaginoplasty outcome in male-to-female transsexuals', *Journal of Sex & Marital Therapy*, 13(4): 265–75. DOI: 10.1080/00926238708403899

Blickensderfer, K., McCormick, B., Myers, J., Goodwin, I., Agarwal, C., Horns, J. (2023) 'Gender-affirming vaginoplasty and vulvoplasty: an initial experience', *Urology*, 76: 232–6. DOI: 10.1016/j.urology.2023.03.002

Bloemen, E.M., Rosen, T., LoFaso, V.M., Lasky, A., Church, S., Hall, P. et al (2019) 'Lesbian, gay, bisexual, and transgender older adults' experiences with elder abuse and neglect', *Journal of the American Geriatrics Society*, 67(11): 2338–45. DOI: 10.1111/jgs.16101

Boas, S.R., Ascha, M., Morrison, S.D., Massie, J.P., Nolan, I.T., Shen, J.K. et al (2019) 'Outcomes and predictors of revision labiaplasty and clitoroplasty after gender-affirming genital surgery', *Plastic and Reconstructive Surgery*, 144(6): 1451–61. DOI: 10.1097/PRS.0000000000006282

Boskey, E.R., Mehra, G., Jolly, D. and Ganor, O. (2022) 'Concerns about internal erectile prostheses among transgender men who have undergone phalloplasty', *The Journal of Sexual Medicine*, 19(6): 1055–9. DOI: 10.1016/j.jsxm.2022.03.604

Buncamper, M.E., van der Sluis, W.B., van der Pas, R.S.D., Özer, M., Smit, J.M., Witte, B.I. et al (2016) 'Surgical outcome after penile inversion vaginoplasty: a retrospective study of 475 transgender women', *Plastic and Reconstructive Surgery*, 138(5): 999–1007. DOI: 10.1097/PRS.0000000000002684

Butler, R.N. (1969) 'Age-ism: another form of bigotry', *The Gerontologist*, 9(4): 243–6. DOI: 10.1093/geront/9.4_part_1.243

Castle, E.R., Blasdel, G., Robinson, I.S., Zhao, L.C. and Bluebond-Langner, R. (2022) 'A comparison of non-surgical methods used by phalloplasty and metoidioplasty patients to improve connection to genitals: how usage of methods and their perceived helpfulness shift after surgery', World Professional Association of Transgender Health 27th Scientific Symposium Surgeon's Only Programme, September.

Catlett, L., Acquaviva, K.D., Campbell, L., Ducar, D., Page, E.H., Patton, J. et al (2023) 'End-of-life care for transgender older adults', *Global Qualitative Nursing Research*, 10: 23333936231161130. DOI: 10.1177/23333936231161128

Chang, S.C., Singh, A.A. and dickey, l.m. (2018) *A Clinician's Guide to Gender-Affirming Care: Working with Transgender and Gender Nonconforming Clients*, np: New Harbinger Publications, Available from: https://play.google.com/store/books/details?id=feFiDwAAQBAJ

Cipolletta, S., Votadoro, R. and Faccio, E. (2017) 'Online support for transgender people: an analysis of forums and social networks', *Health & Social Care in the Community*, 25(5): 1542–51. DOI: 10.1111/hsc.12448

Crenshaw, K. (1989) 'Demarginalizing the intersection of race and sex: a Black feminist critique of antidiscrimination doctrine, feminist theory and antiracist politics', *University of Chicago Legal Forum*, 1989(1): 139–67, Available from: https://chicagounbound.uchicago.edu/cgi/viewcontent.cgi?article=1052&context=uclf

Cui, P., Wang, S., Wang, P., Yang, L., Kong, C. and Lu, S. (2022) 'Comparison of perioperative outcomes in frail patients following multilevel lumbar fusion surgery with and without the implementation of the enhanced recovery after surgery protocol', *Frontiers in Surgery*, 9: 997657. DOI: 10.3389/fsurg.2022.997657

Davis, L.J. (ed) (2016) *The Disability Studies Reader* (5th edn), New York: Routledge. DOI: 10.4324/9781315680668/disability-studies-reader-lennard-davis

De Cuypere, G., T'Sjoen, G., Beerten, R., Selvaggi, G., De Sutter, P., Hoebeke, P. et al (2005) 'Sexual and physical health after sex reassignment surgery', *Archives of Sexual Behavior*, 34(6): 679–90. DOI: 10.1007/s10508-005-7926-5

DeLamater, J. and Plante, R.F. (eds) (2015) *Handbook of the Sociology of Sexualities*, Heidelberg: Springer, Available from: https://play.google.com/store/books/details?id=0d3yCQAAQBAJ

Denny, D. (2002) 'A selective bibliography of transsexualism', *Journal of Gay & Lesbian Psychotherapy*, 6(2): 35–66. DOI: 10.1300/J236v06n02_04

Donato, D.P., Walzer, N.K., Rivera, A., Wright, L. and Agarwal, C.A. (2017) 'Female-to-male chest reconstruction: a review of technique and outcomes', *Annals of Plastic Surgery*, 79(3): 259–63. DOI: 10.1097/SAP.0000000000001099

Finlayson, E.V.A. and Birkmeyer, J.D. (2001) 'Operative mortality', *Effective Clinical Practice: ECP*, 4(4): 172–7, Available from: https://www.researchgate.net/publication/11820969

Frederick, M.J., Berhanu, A.E. and Bartlett, R. (2017) 'Chest surgery in female to male transgender individuals', *Annals of Plastic Surgery*, 78(3): 249–53. DOI: 10.1097/SAP.0000000000000882

Fredriksen-Goldsen, K.I., Cook-Daniels, L., Kim, H.-J., Erosheva, E.A., Emlet, C.A., Hoy-Ellis, C.P. et al (2014) 'Physical and mental health of transgender older adults: an at-risk and underserved population', *The Gerontologist*, 54(3): 488–500. DOI: 10.1093/geront/gnt021

Gaither, T.W., Awad, M.A., Osterberg, E.C., Murphy, G.P., Romero, A., Bowers, M.L. (2018) 'Postoperative complications following primary penile inversion vaginoplasty among 330 male-to-female transgender patients', *The Journal of Urology*, 199(3): 760–5. DOI: 10.1016/j.juro.2017.10.013

Gamble, R.M., Taylor, S.S., Huggins, A.D. and Ehrenfeld, J.M. (2020) 'Trans-specific Geriatric Health Assessment (TGHA): an inclusive clinical guideline for the geriatric transgender patient in a primary care setting', *Maturitas*, 132: 70–5. DOI: 10.1016/j.maturitas.2019.12.005

George, A., Janardhana, N. and Muralidhar, D. (2015) 'Quality of life of transgender older adults', *International Journal of Humanities and Social Science Invention*, 4(6): 7–11, Available from: https://www.ijhssi.org/papers/v4(6)/Version-2/B046207011.pdf

Goddard, J.C., Vickery, R.M., Qureshi, A., Summerton, D.J., Khoosal, D. and Terry, T.R. (2007) 'Feminizing genitoplasty in adult transsexuals: early and long-term surgical results', *BJU International*, 100(3): 607–13. DOI: 10.1111/j.1464-410X.2007.07017.x

Goins, R.T., Williams, K.A., Carter, M.W., Spencer, M. and Solovieva, T. (2005) 'Perceived barriers to health care access among rural older adults: a qualitative study', *The Journal of Rural Health: Official Journal of the American Rural Health Association and the National Rural Health Care Association*, 21(3): 206–13. DOI: 10.1111/j.1748-0361.2005.tb00084.x

Greenwood, N., Menzies-Gow, E., Nilsson, D., Aubrey, D., Emery, C.L. and Richardson, A. (2018) 'Experiences of older people dying in nursing homes: a narrative systematic review of qualitative studies', *BMJ Open*, 8(6): e021285. DOI: 10.1136/bmjopen-2017-021285

Grenier, A. and Hanley, J. (2007) 'Older women and "frailty": aged, gendered and embodied resistance', *Current Sociology/La Sociologie contemporaine*, 55(2): 211–28. DOI: 10.1177/0011392107073303

Hargittai, E., Piper, A.M. and Morris, M.R. (2019) 'From internet access to internet skills: digital inequality among older adults', *Universal Access in the Information Society*, 18(4): 881–90. DOI: 10.1007/s10209-018-0617-5

Harner, V. (2021) 'Trans intracommunity support & knowledge sharing in the United States & Canada: a scoping literature review', *Health & Social Care in the Community*, 29(6): 1715–28. DOI: 10.1111/hsc.13276

Hatzenbuehler, M.L., Phelan, J.C. and Link, B.G. (2013) 'Stigma as a fundamental cause of population health inequalities', *American Journal of Public Health*, 103(5): 813–21. DOI: 10.2105/AJPH.2012.301069

Holzapfel, S. (1994) 'Aging and sexuality', *Canadian Family Physician/Medecin de famille canadien*, 40: 748–50, 753–4, 757–8, passim, Available from: https://www.ncbi.nlm.nih.gov/pubmed/8199527

Javier, N.M. (2019) 'Geriatric transgender care', in L. Poretsky and W.C. Hembree (eds) *Transgender Medicine*, Cham: Springer International, pp 93–112. DOI: 10.1007/978-3-030-05683-4_6

Kaye, H.S., Harrington, C. and LaPlante, M.P. (2010) 'Long-term care: who gets it, who provides it, who pays, and how much?', *Health Affairs*, 29(1): 11–21. DOI: 10.1377/hlthaff.2009.0535

Kehlet, H. (1997) 'Multimodal approach to control postoperative pathophysiology and rehabilitation', *British Journal of Anaesthesia*, 78(5): 606–17. DOI: 10.1093/bja/78.5.606

Kennis, M., Duecker, F., T'Sjoen, G., Sack, A.T. and Dewitte, M. (2022) 'Gender affirming medical treatment desire and treatment motives in binary and non-binary transgender individuals', *The Journal of Sexual Medicine*, 19(7): 1173–84. DOI: 10.1016/j.jsxm.2022.03.603

Klein, A. and Golub, S.A. (2020) 'Enhancing gender-affirming provider communication to increase health care access and utilization among transgender men and trans-masculine non-binary individuals', *LGBT Health*, 7(6): 292–304. DOI: 10.1089/lgbt.2019.0294

Klein, A. and Golub, S.A. (2022a) 'Ethical HIV research with transgender and non-binary communities in the United States', *Journal of the International AIDS Society*, 25(suppl 5): e25971. DOI: 10.1002/jia2.25971

Klein, A. and Golub, S.A. (2022b) 'Nothing about us without us: building patient-centered outcomes research capacity in a national consortium of LGBTQ+ health centers', Hunter Alliance for Research & Translation (HART).

Kloer, C., Blasdel, G., Shakir, N., Parker, A., Gómez, A.I., Zhao, L.C. et al (2023) 'Does genital self-image correspond with sexual health before and after vaginoplasty?', *Plastic and Reconstructive Surgery: Global Open*, 11(2): e4806. DOI: 10.1097/GOX.0000000000004806

Li, J., Zhao, F., Gao, J., Dong, W., Yu, X., Zhu, C. et al (2023) 'Enhanced recovery after surgery (ERAS) protocol in geriatric patients underwent unicompartmental knee arthroplasty: a retrospective cohort study', *Medicine*, 102(6): e32941. DOI: 10.1097/MD.0000000000032941

Martínez-Escribano, C., Arteaga Moreno, F., Peredo, D.C., Gonzalez, F.J.B., De la Cámara-de las Heras, J.M. and Tarazona Santabalbina, F.J. (2022) 'Before-and-after study of the first four years of the Enhanced Recovery after Surgery (ERAS®) programme in older adults undergoing elective colorectal cancer surgery', *International Journal of Environmental Research and Public Health*, 19(22): 15299. DOI: 10.3390/ijerph192215299

Massie, J.P., Morrison, S.D., van Maasdam, J. and Satterwhite, T. (2018) 'Predictors of patient satisfaction and postoperative complications in penile inversion vaginoplasty', *Plastic and Reconstructive Surgery*, 141(6): 911e–921e. DOI: 10.1097/PRS.0000000000004427

McCann, K. (1990) 'AIDS in the nineties: from science to policy; care in the community and by the community', *AIDS Care*, 2(4): 421–4. DOI: 10.1080/09540129008257767

McCrone, S. (2018) 'LGBT healthcare disparities, discrimination, and societal stigma: the mental and physical health risks related to sexual and/or gender minority status', *American Journal of Medical Research*, 5(1): 91–6, Available from: https://www.ceeol.com/content-files/document-661121.pdf

Meyerowitz, J.J. (2009) *How Sex Changed*, Cambridge, MA: Harvard University Press, Available from: https://play.google.com/store/books/details?id=XFP2PmYPBBAC

Monstrey, S., Selvaggi, G., Ceulemans, P., van Landuyt, K., Bowman, C., Blondeel, P. et al (2008) 'Chest-wall contouring surgery in female-to-male transsexuals: a new algorithm', *Plastic and Reconstructive Surgery*, 121(3): 849–59. DOI: 10.1097/01.prs.0000299921.15447.b2

Pang, C., Gutman, G. and de Vries, B. (2019) 'Later life care planning and concerns of transgender older adults in Canada', *International Journal of Aging & Human Development*, 89(1): 39–56. DOI: 10.1177/0091415019843520

Pereira, H. and Banerjee, D. (2021) 'Successful aging among older LGBTQIA+ people: future research and implications', *Frontiers in Psychiatry*, 12: 756649. DOI: 10.3389/fpsyt.2021.756649

Pittelkow, E.M., Duquette, S.P., Rhamani, F., Rogers, C. and Gallagher, S. (2020) 'Female-to-male gender-confirming drainless mastectomy may be safe in obese males', *Aesthetic Surgery Journal*, 40(3): NP85–NP93. DOI: 10.1093/asj/sjz335

Poteat, T., German, D. and Kerrigan, D. (2013) 'Managing uncertainty: a grounded theory of stigma in transgender health care encounters', *Social Science & Medicine*, 84: 22–9. DOI: 10.1016/j.socscimed.2013.02.019

Preto, M., Blecher, G., Timpano, M., Gontero, P. and Falcone, M. (2020) 'The frontier of penile implants in phalloplasty: is the ZSI 475 FTM what we have been waiting for?', *International Journal of Impotence Research*, 33(7): 779–83. DOI: 10.1038/s41443-020-00396-2

Puckett, J.A., Cleary, P., Rossman, K., Newcomb, M.E. and Mustanski, B. (2018) 'Barriers to gender-affirming care for transgender and gender nonconforming individuals', *Sexuality Research & Social Policy*, 15(1): 48–59. DOI: 10.1007/s13178-017-0295-8

Purohit, R.S., Kent, M. and Djordjevic, M.L. (2022) 'Penile prosthesis in transgender men after phalloplasty', *Indian Journal of Plastic Surgery*, 55(2): 168–73. DOI: 10.1055/s-0041-1740523

Robinson, I.S., Blasdel, G., Cohen, O., Zhao, L.C. and Bluebond-Langner, R. (2021) 'Surgical outcomes following gender affirming penile reconstruction: patient-reported outcomes from a multi-center, international survey of 129 transmasculine patients', *The Journal of Sexual Medicine*, 18(4): 800–11. DOI: 10.1016/j.jsxm.2021.01.183

Rosen, R.C. (1996) 'Erectile dysfunction: the medicalization of male sexuality', *Clinical Psychology Review*, 16(6): 497–519. DOI: 10.1016/0272-7358(96)00032-3

Rossi Neto, R., Hintz, F., Krege, S., Rubben, H. and vom Dorp, F. (2012) 'Gender reassignment surgery: a 13 year review of surgical outcomes', *International Brazilian Journal of Urology*, 38(1): 97–107. DOI: 10.1590/s1677-55382012000100014

Shih, K., de Oliveira Jr, G.S., Qin, C. and Kim, J.Y. (2015) 'The impact of advancing age on postoperative outcomes in plastic surgery', *Journal of Plastic, Reconstructive & Aesthetic Surgery*, 68(11): 1610–15. DOI: 10.1016/j.bjps.2015.07.015

Shiu, C., Muraco, A. and Fredriksen-Goldsen, K. (2016) 'Invisible care: friend and partner care among older lesbian, gay, bisexual, and transgender (LGBT) adults', *Journal of the Society for Social Work and Research*, 7(3): 527–46. DOI: 10.1086/687325

shuster, s.m. (2021) *Trans Medicine: The Emergence and Practice of Treating Gender*, New York: NYU Press, Available from: https://play.google.com/store/books/details?id=pHwDEAAAQBAJ

Skorochod, R., Rysin, R. and Wolf, Y. (2023) 'Age-related outcomes of chest masculinization surgery: a single-surgeon retrospective cohort study', *Plastic and Reconstructive Surgery: Global Open*, 11(2): e4799. DOI: 10.1097/GOX.0000000000004799

Sorg, H., Sorg, C.G.G., Tilkorn, D.J., Thönnes, S., Karimo, R. and Hauser, J. (2023) 'Free flaps for skin and soft tissue reconstruction in the elderly patient: indication or contraindication', *Medical Sciences*, 11(1). DOI: 10.3390/medsci11010012

Stryker, S. (2009) *Transgender History*, np: Da Capo Press, Available from: https://play.google.com/store/books/details?id=kEfZ1knAguMC

Timmermans, F.W., Elfering, L., Steensma, T.D., Bouman, M.-B. and van der Sluis W.B. (2023) 'Mastectomy is a safe procedure in transgender men with a history of breast reduction', *Journal of Plastic Surgery and Hand Surgery*, 57(1–6): 483–7. DOI: 10.1080/2000656X.2022.2164293

Towler, L.B., Graham, C.A., Bishop, F.L. and Hinchliff, S. (2021) 'Older adults' embodied experiences of aging and their perceptions of societal stigmas toward sexuality in later life', *Social Science & Medicine*, 287: 114355. DOI: 10.1016/j.socscimed.2021.114355

Townsend, N.T. and Robinson, T.N. (2015) 'Surgical risk and comorbidity in older urologic patients', *Clinics in Geriatric Medicine*, 31(4): 591–601. DOI: 10.1016/j.cger.2015.06.009

Waling, A., Lyons, A., Alba, B., Minichiello, V., Barrett, C., Hughes, M. et al (2020) 'Trans women's perceptions of residential aged care in Australia', *British Journal of Social Work*, 50(5): 1304–23. DOI: 10.1093/bjsw/bcz122

Waling, A., Lyons, A., Alba, B., Minichiello, V., Barrett, C., Hughes, M. et al (2022) 'Experiences of informal caregiving among older lesbian and gay adults in Australia', *Australasian Journal on Ageing*, 41(3): 424–30. DOI: 10.1111/ajag.13076

Wang, L.C. and Poppas, D.P. (2017) 'Surgical outcomes and complications of reconstructive surgery in the female congenital adrenal hyperplasia patient: what every endocrinologist should know', *The Journal of Steroid Biochemistry and Molecular Biology*, 165(Pt A): 137–44. DOI: 10.1016/j.jsbmb.2016.03.021

Watt, J., Tricco, A.C., Talbot-Hamon, C., Pham, B., Rios, P., Grudniewicz, A. et al (2018) 'Identifying older adults at risk of harm following elective surgery: a systematic review and meta-analysis', *BMC Medicine*, 16(1): 2. DOI: 10.1186/s12916-017-0986-2

Wicke, C., Bachinger, A., Coerper, S., Beckert, S., Witte, M.B. and Königsrainer, A. (2009) 'Aging influences wound healing in patients with chronic lower extremity wounds treated in a specialized wound care center', *Wound Repair and Regeneration*, 17(1): 25–33. DOI: 10.1111/j.1524-475X.2008.00438.x

Wolf, Y. and Kwartin, S. (2021) 'Classification of transgender man's breast for optimizing chest masculinizing gender-affirming surgery', *Plastic and Reconstructive Surgery: Global Open*, 9(1): e3363. DOI: 10.1097/GOX.0000000000003363

World Health Organization (2021) 'Ageing: ageism', Available from: https://www.who.int/news-room/questions-and-answers/item/ageing-ageism

Xue, Q.-L. (2011) 'The frailty syndrome: definition and natural history', *Clinics in Geriatric Medicine*, 27(1): 1–15. DOI: 10.1016/j.cger.2010.08.009

9

What is being done to support trans older people facing intimate and domestic abuse?

Trish Hafford-Letchfield and Keira McCormack

Introduction

The stigma, discrimination and violence faced by trans people globally is pervasive and well documented (Arayasirikul et al, 2022). While there is growing appreciation of intimate partner violence (IPV) and domestic abuse (DA) in relationships for lesbian, gay and bisexual (LGB) populations, trans people are a group of 'hidden victims' and there is very little literature on their experiences (Gelles, 1997, p 96). The dearth of empirical work and the invisibility of trans people when exploring intimate and familial relationships and the environments in which intimate and domestic violence takes place sits within the broader picture of LGB people being at an elevated risk of IPV (Langenderfer-Magruder et al, 2016; Valentine et al, 2017). This chapter considers what is known about DA and IPV perpetrated against trans people in *later life* alongside any literature on adult safeguarding that might overlap in presentation (Cook-Daniels, 2010). This lack of visibility of older people who are gender diverse, the failure to ask or record gender identity when people are accessing or using support services and/or trans and non-binary individuals' fear of sharing information with professionals and service providers are all contributing factors to the failure of being able to screen, recognise and assess IPV and DA.

This chapter is written from our experience of working in the UK as a trans historied woman and cis woman, one of whom has extensive practice expertise in DA and the other in researching LGBTQ+ later life experience of health and social care. We draw on the sparse but important body of work on trans DA along with some of the broader literature on identity abuse. This is used to articulate what can be learned to support trans people better in later life who have or may be experiencing DA. We first consider what is known about the broader issues of violence against trans people before going on to highlight the types of violence experienced by trans individuals and the settings in which DA and IPV occur. We highlight the epistemological, political and social context for trans DA and look at barriers and challenges in identifying, reporting and responding to DA for trans people in *later life* given the lack of research and practice guidance in health and social care. We then illustrate the barriers they may face in help seeking and summarise the key points for informing improved practice in both prevention and interventions with older trans people with pointers for further research.

We use the following definitions familiar to UK and international audiences:

Domestic Abuse refers to any incident or pattern of incidents of controlling, coercive, threatening behaviour, violence or abuse between those aged 16 or over who are or have been intimate partners or family members regardless of gender or sexuality. (Home Office, 2018, para 1)

Intimate partner violence refers to behaviour within an intimate relationship that causes physical, sexual or psychological harm, including acts of physical aggression, sexual coercion, psychological abuse and controlling behaviours. This definition covers violence by both current and former spouses and partners. (World Health Organization website, nd)

Violence against trans people

The settings where trans and non-binary people experience marginalisation and abuse are of both a private and public nature (Grant et al, 2011). The Trans Murder Monitoring (TMM) research project by TGEU (Transgender Europe) systematically monitors, collects, and analyses reports of homicides of trans and gender diverse people worldwide. Updates of the results are published here: https://transrespect.org/en/research/tmm. Globally, homicides against trans people accounted for 321 trans and gender diverse people who were reported as murdered between 1 October 2022 and 30 September 2023 (Trans Murder Monitoring Global Update, 2023). Nine in ten (96 per cent) of those murdered were trans women, and most victims were Black and migrant trans women of colour and trans sex workers. It is accepted that these numbers are a small glimpse of reality on the ground, where data are not systematically collected. Homicides involving trans victims often go unreported and remain unsolved. However, existing sources point to the significant role of domestic and sexual violence in the reported fatalities (Talusan, 2016; Waters and Yacka-Bible, 2017). Significant to this chapter is that a substantial number of those murdered were killed in their own home: for example, one analysis of reported murders perpetrated against trans women in Latin America found that 78.8 per cent of murders occurred at home (Silva et al, 2022).

Trans individuals are twice as likely to be assaulted throughout their lives compared to cis individuals and are particularly likely to be subject to sexual violence and IPV (Brown and Herman, 2015; Swan et al, 2021). Specific to the UK, a small-scale survey (n = 71) found that almost half of respondents (46 per cent) claimed that they had previously experienced transphobic IPV (Scottish Transgender Alliance, 2008). Another independent UK based survey identified 14 per cent trans victim/survivors of which 12 per cent were 50 years or older which although fewer in number, respondents over-reported the highest levels of abuse across all types (Magić and Kelley, 2018). Trans women are five times more likely to be sexually abused when compared to cis women (Smith et al, 2017), and verbal, psychological and physical aggression towards trans women is also highly common in Western societies (Flentje et al, 2016). Other research with trans samples has found that younger people are more likely to experience more recent sexual and physical violence than older people (Cook-Daniels and Munson, 2010; Sterzing et al, 2019) but this finding does not consider that those who are older will have had cumulative opportunities for victimisation to occur (Messinger et al, 2022). Messinger and colleagues' (2022) secondary data analysis conducted with 15,198 transgender IPV survivors from the 2015 'U.S. transgender survey' noted that 55 per cent of the sample reported experiencing at least one type of IPV in their lifetime. However, only 2.1 per cent of the respondents were 65 years and over. Among those who did not seek help, as the age of respondents increased, their likelihood of reporting decreased significantly for fear of transphobic response. Those living with disabilities that are known to increase or cumulate in later life may lead to a person to become more dependent on a significant other or become dependent in the care system, which could make them a vulnerable target for harm. Messinger et al suggest that more research is needed to understand this finding and to conceptualise lifetime measures of IPV (2022, p 18828).

A cross-sectional study of 121 trans people (71 per cent were trans women) in Brazil in 2019–20 (Pexioto et al, 2022) investigated the associations between self-reported 'passing'[1] and different forms of IPV. While the concept of passing is a contentious area given the burden it places on trans people of unrealistic gender standards, in this study passing resulted in higher rates of family violence as well as lower rates of observed police violence and violence in open and closed public spaces. The implication is that people who are visibly trans (or otherwise perceived as gender non-conforming) are likely to experience stranger violence and police violence, whereas those who are perceived as (more often) women, experience family and intimate violence.

While less is known about the experience of trans individuals at the intersection of gender and ageing, Hillman (2020) examined lifetime prevalence of IPV and its association with health among trans adults through secondary data analysis of responses from 3,462 trans adults aged 50 and older in the United States. Analysis revealed significant differences among the percentage of trans adults aged 50 and older who reported lifetime experience with trans-specific (41 per cent), physical (36 per cent), psychological (30 per cent), severe physical (24 per cent), stalking (12 per cent) and sexual (10 per cent) IPV (p 215). The largest group (41 per cent) experienced partner abuse that specifically targeted their trans identity, whereas the smallest group experienced stalking and sexual abuse. Hillman also identified poor health-related outcomes involving substance use and poor mental health among trans adults in later life. Those who had experienced IPV reported that they were significantly more likely to view their current general health more negatively (p 220). The effects from IPV on suicide, depressive or traumatic symptoms are well known (Johns et al, 2018).

Trans people living with disabilities report higher rates of DA and IPV (James et al, 2016). These may be compounded by the cumulative effects of everyday transphobia in later life as demonstrated in other chapters of this book. For cis people in later life, negative outcomes associated with IPV include increased rates of hospitalisation, disability, nursing home placement and a 300 per cent increase in mortality (Dong et al, 2009; Breiding and Armour, 2015; Warmling et al, 2017). Further, as Westwood (2019) points out, systematic reviews of the literature on 'elder abuse' make not a single reference to sexual or gender identity, not even to highlight their absence in research. Therefore, the (unknown) consequences for trans people are likely to be more significant in relation to vulnerabilities at the intersection of age, disability, abuse and gender identity. While there is little research on the long-term physical and psychological impact of transphobic violence, coping strategies and resilience among trans people in later life (see Toze's Chapter 3), it is reasonable to assume that this will also be a significant source of trauma. Not least, given what we do know from the research findings is that most trans adults are extremely fearful of residential care where they may be exposed to both physical and psychological violence (Witten, 2014; Willis et al, 2021). Westwood (2019) uses the concept of polyvictimisation in her intersectional and feminist analysis of power relations of the literature on LGBT elder abuse. She articulates how different forms of harm spill into each other, compounding their impact on a person in later life and increasing the risk to their physical and mental wellbeing (p 99).

The epistemological, political and social context for trans DA

Scholars, activists and survivors have described heightened vulnerabilities to domestic and sexual violence among LGBT+ people as rooted in social, political and economic conditions that systematically devalue and diminish their lives and relationships (Ristock, 2011). A common theme in the literature is the idea that the DA movement has lost its strong political foundation as services are delivered from within the mainstream (heteronormative and cisnormative) framework for social care provision (Rogers, 2016). Brown and Herman (2015) suggests that 'perpetrators are acutely aware of the individual and institutional vulnerabilities faced by trans people and these vulnerabilities feature explicitly in the abuse tactics and harm done' (p 117).

Cisgenderism provides a framework that can help to articulate trans people's experiences of DA in micro-level settings (that is, within and across personal relationships) as well as in relation to macro-level influences (for example, social and cultural norms; Rogers, 2021, p 2090). In short, most DA studies are rooted in a gender paradigm which positions men as perpetrators and women as victims (Rogers, 2017), and this public notion can be seen to invisibilise, silence and invalidate trans and non-binary people's experiences. If DA is conceptualised as hetero- and gender normative, it reinforces a systemic practice and epistemological erasure of trans people and their experiences (Serano, 2007). Further, public records and population-level surveys echo and reproduce dominant social ideologies of sex and gender that treat 'males/men' and 'females/women' as cohesive and mutually exclusive categories (Namaste, 2000).

These are important points for DA services in how they present to trans and non-binary older individuals and how active they are in supporting access and ongoing provision. Within the UK, at the time of writing, this has become an overly sensitive and divisive topic which takes no account of ageing. As 'gender reassignment' is a protected characteristic under the Equality Act (UK Government, 2010), there is provision for trans women to be treated the same as any other woman and with the right to access women-only spaces and services. However, the Equality and Human Rights Commission (EHRC) has stated that trans people can be legitimately excluded from single-sex space or services if the reasons are 'justifiable and proportionate' for reasons of privacy, decency, to prevent trauma or to ensure health and safety (EHRC, 2022, p 6). Those with a Gender Recognition Certificate (GRC) can be excluded as a 'proportionate means of achieving a legitimate aim' (p 7). It is important to note that DA support services are one of the areas named as one area for justification. The case in the UK courts in 2021 brought by the Authentic Equity Alliance (AEA) (a community interest company established in 2018 to promote the personal and professional development of women and girls) challenged whether some aspects of the EHRC guidance were lawful (*AEA v EHRC*, 2021). The judge decided that this should not be put in front of the courts given that the EHRC guidance is intended as a summary rather than detailed legal analysis. However, during the arguments, the judge commented that gender 'appearance' was relevant, and the EHRC agreed that women-only space does not have to include anyone who is male at birth. They also described prescriptive inclusion policies along the lines of self-ID as being 'directly inconsistent' with their Code of Practice. The judge strongly agreed with the EHRC that a better challenge would have been brought by an individual service user against an individual service provider, rather than in the abstract at the level of the EHRC and the AEA as this case did. However, this was not a good outcome for different groups using DA support services, who tend to be overstretched and ill positioned to sustain lengthy legal battles. Further, this makes progressive policies and service provision challenging for service providers who are not conversant with trans human rights and advocacy.

Therefore, the debate remains on what is justified and proportionate, particularly from those who wish to be able to exclude trans people without needing to demonstrate proportionality. In the context of media controversy, a significant upsurge in public anti-trans sentiment and the impact of gender critical feminists debate on gender identities have all contributed to a political landscape of anti-trans politics, especially in Western societies (Pearce et al, 2020). For older people who have lived through a history of transgressed human rights, including participation in the feminist movement, this repositioning of them as being a threat to cis women's safety may undermine their own rights to safety and help seeking.

Rogers' (2021) UK empirical research of people with experiences of DA illustrated different forms of cisgenderism, namely embodiment and identity abuse, intersectionality and identity abuse, misgendering, and pathologising. Asserting that 'identity abuse' is a form of DA which uses gender normative and cisgenderist ideas and beliefs to denigrate, coerce and control, Rogers illuminates the extensive ways in which cisgenderism can be operationalised through the practices of partners and family members within intimate and familial relationships with trans people. Rogers' (2017) earlier conceptualisation of transphobic abuse as 'honour'-based abuse also offers a novel way of exploring and conceptualising trans people's experiences of family-based abuse and for understanding other relational contexts, for example the embarrassment/shame that a family sometimes express at having a trans person in the family. For people in later life, this shame might extend to having a trans parent or grandparent in the family. Gender is a dichotomous social construct embedded and regulated in a patriarchal power structure (Guadalupe-Diaz and Jasinski, 2017), which requires an analysis of situational power that frames the experiences of abuse for trans victim/survivors.

Recognising and identifying domestic abuse in later life

Expanding our limited knowledge of DA among trans adults in later life is essential to the provision of trans-inclusive and accessible services. Within research, this includes but is not restricted to:

- threats to 'out' or disclose an individual's gender diversity status (Cook-Daniels, 2015), specifically against trans men (Forge, 2013) and women in relationships with cis men (Jauk, 2013);
- telling people they are mentally ill and blaming people for making the life of a loved one harder;
- psychological bullying, for example by saying that you "are not a 'real' women or man", you do not look like or are believable as men/women (Cook-Daniels, 2015);
- undermining identities by refusing to use the correct name and pronouns;
- telling individuals that 'real men' enjoy rough sex, do not cry or would not report abuse and taking advantage of the lack of structural support for gender identity and expression;
- isolating and eroding trans individuals' sense of self by making them feel less than human or undeserving of love (Cook and Daniels, 2015) and/or not being 'trans enough' (Bornstein et al, 2006);
- withholding or destroying clothing, prescription medication (James et al, 2016) and other personal items such as chest binders or make-up that are associated with gender identity (Hillman, 2020);
- causing damage or mutilation to parts of the individual's body or person, for example the chest, genitals, head and body hair (White and Goldberg, 2006);
- purposefully causing dysphoria through inappropriate touching or using offensive terminology about a person's body (FORGE, 2013);
- outright refusing to acknowledge a trans person's gender identity or monitoring or scrutinising a trans person's gender expression (Cook-Daniels and Munson, 2010);
- lack of respect for the gendered self that people may have fought for recognition across their lifetime (Willis et al, 2021);
- within long-term care environments, older trans individuals can be especially hindered from exercising everyday choices over dress and presentation, with increasing reliance on care workers to support this (Hudson, 2011). They can lose their gendered self that they have fought for recognition across their lifetime (Willis et al, 2021);
- individual gaslighting and manipulation (Guadalupe-Diaz and Jasinski, 2016) within interpersonal relationships for dependent people with health issues associated with ageing – such as being told that one is losing cognitive capacity, or that their ageing bodies are unattractive;
- institutional gaslighting and manipulation through ignoring or silencing trans people's differences in care settings or using difference to exclude them from relationships, resources and trans-related care;
- actively preventing access to gender-affirming medical treatment, support spaces or information. In care settings, examples including ignorance and omission can result in not signposting, advocating or making referrals, or dismissing someone's desires and choices that affirm their gender

identity. Professionals assuming and advising people they are too old, not fit enough or challenging their entitlement to resources that support gender affirmation and being obstructive in the access or use of those resources where a person can't do this independently;
- using trans identity as grounds to contest parental or family rights (Hafford-Letchfield et al, 2018) or to discredit witness statements in courts and with law enforcement, advocates, family members and friends, and other potential interveners (Bornstein et al, 2006; Guadalupe-Diaz and Anthony, 2017);
- asserting that being trans makes you 'public' property and gives people the right to ask personal questions which can add to an older trans person's vulnerability, making IPV/DA easier to perpetuate. Trans older individuals in their own homes may be asked inappropriate questions about their bodies or clothes during personal care or be subject to expressions of disapproval or disgust and asked to justify their needs for gender-affirming care.

Social isolation is particularly concerning for trans women of colour, who may already experience social or family exclusion because of their gender or sexuality identity, for some compounded by isolation resulting from migration Hawkey et al, 2012). Sharing reflections on running a peer support group for trans people, Schultz (2020) reported how easy it can be for individuals to succumb to fear and paranoia, particularly with knowledge that they are statistically likely to be assaulted. This can reduce people's everyday behaviour so it is not seen to invite violence, expecting violence or sexual assault and where IPV may seem par for the course. Shultz comments that 'in community spaces, we speak of assault casually and we tell of our rapes and then say, "whatever"' (2020, p 145). As discussed by Toze in Chapter 3, there is a lack of dedicated peer-support space for older trans people and few such groups. All-age groups in both trans and DA may be much less experienced in responding to IPV experienced by older people.

More broadly, social and structural inequities increase situational vulnerabilities to violence for trans people, such as high rates of housing insecurity and homelessness, economic discrimination, reliance on survival sex and poor conditions in sex work, disability and incarceration (Spade, 2015; James et al, 2016; Kattari and Begun, 2017). All these factors illustrate the pervasiveness of social stigma and how structural exclusions may be uniquely leveraged as a tactic of IPV.

Barriers to help seeking

Older trans individuals are especially at risk of partner victimisation due to shame, isolation or loneliness, which may lower relationship expectations and make them vulnerable to staying in harmful relationships (Brown, 2011). Other older people pride themselves on self-reliance and may be hesitant to rely on others for help. They may find it difficult to identify abuse and/or relevant community resources (Bornstein et al, 2006). As illustrated by Schultz's observations earlier, trans people accept what they are used to and may be afraid of not being believed or being influenced by what they thought others expected to see of an IPV victim versus their own lived experience (Brown, 2011, p 783). For older people, this can enhance the emotional and psychological impacts of rejection, and being belittled, dismissed and invalidated can be further complicated by internalised ageism. Guadalupe-Diaz and Jansen (2017) identified two major themes in the help-seeking process by trans survivors of IPV. These were what they termed as 'walking the gender tightrope' (p 782), in which participants first struggled with gendered notions of victimisation that made it difficult to identify abuse, and second the challenges of 'navigating genderist resources' (p 784).

For older people, having a reduced income and an increased reliance on a partner or other person for care (Beaulaurier et al, 2005; Messinger et al, 2022) can reduce help seeking. A low income is known to be a cumulative factor for trans people experiencing unemployment or having to take low-paid jobs in their earlier life associated with transphobia (Schilt and Wiswall, 2008). Economic stressors may delay retirement. Individuals may also fear being transferred to a care or nursing home (Seelman et al, 2017) or delay accessing those resources that prevent entering long-term care based on fear of discriminatory abuse in their own home by professionals and carers. There is evidence of trans people being exposed to discrimination, both from IPV survivor service providers and aging-related service providers (Messinger et al, 2022; Willis et al, 2021). As suggested earlier, trying to remain unseen in public spaces denies personal visibility or the fostering of a positive self-identity and embodiment, which plays a key role in self-esteem, wellbeing, avoidance of distress and thus active help seeking (Hawkey et al, 2021). Remaining unseen may become less feasible with age or when one becomes less independent. Having to rely on carers and reveal one's body for both intimate personal care and gender-affirming expression in both home and institutional settings can be survivors. Being estranged from their family of origin can leave trans and gender diverse people without support if DA occurs. Further, a person may feel unable to leave an abusive relationship if they have nowhere to take their companion animals (Taylor et al, 2016), which are often a valued source of support for people in later life experiencing loneliness.

Barriers to accessing services

Bornstein et al (2006) noted that for many trans people, shelters are unwelcoming, especially if they require disclosure of trans status or require gender segregation. This is a practice that fails to recognise the needs of gender diverse people (Parry and O'Neal, 2015). One of Rogers' (2016, p 71) participants said

> 'I would feel neither safe nor comfortable approaching a social care agency which deals with domestic abuse … I do not feel that the agencies providing this type of support are yet at a point where they are willing and committed to engaging with trans people and learning about what type of support we need.' (Max, genderqueer)

Max is referring to the issue of ignorance of trans issues in care services and their lack of community engagement. The rise of gender critical trans-exclusionary feminist arguments against trans women's access to women-only (or sex-segregated, or single-sex) spaces in the UK and elsewhere (Zanghellini, 2020) has also introduced modes of argument making shelters and other safe spaces a hostile setting for trans people. Just one bad referral or experience can erode trust and rapport with an individual survivor and reverberate within interconnected social networks (Jordan et al, 2020). This occurs through explicit exclusion and its discriminatory impacts and primarily in the context of gender-based service models (Jordan et al, 2020, p 540). The popular use of gendered language and imagery in agency materials, websites, shelter spaces and gender-specific services such as women's shelters can reinforce perceptions that such resources are reserved for cis (not trans) women. There are uncertainties and dilemmas for trans men and non-binary people, who effectively must make a choice between misgendering their self to access support or not getting support. They are not then identified because they feel obliged to disguise their trans status.

In the absence of explicit language or clues that trans people will be welcomed, survivors may anticipate additional scrutiny, judgement or rejection and opt to bypass them entirely. Interactions with the police also feature strongly. For example, negative police encounters, including profiling and harassment, deter trans survivors from pursuing law enforcement and other legal interventions (Guadalupe-Diaz and Jasinski, 2017). This is compounded for trans people of colour who fear being mistreated as a victim (Jordan et al, 2020). This is in the wider context of poor conviction rates for IPV/DA, a fear of confirming an inaccurate stereotype of trans people as predators (Guadalupe-Diaz and Jasinski, 2017) or making the trans community look bad or worse (Cook-Daniels, 2015). Our practice observation is that trans women are perceived as essentially 'male' and capable of defending or looking after themselves in common with cis male victims. They may be less believed or seen as the perpetrator in a counter-allegation given the legacy of 'trans panic' defence cases. Jordan and colleagues' (2020) qualitative study summarises these barriers through five interconnected themes related to ongoing inequalities for trans survivors of IPV: (1) fear of and resistance to using the criminal legal system, (2) exclusions from gender-based programmes, (3) the limited impact of compliance and competency approaches to inclusion, (4) advocacy practices focused on a single source of violence and (5) the diversion to and overburdening of LGBTQ programmes. It has also been noted that when structural and formal resources are inaccessible, unwelcoming and discriminatory, families and friendships become much more important (Guadalupe-Diaz and Jasinski, 2017).

Structural barriers

Age is an especially crucial factor in help seeking (Donovan et al, 2006), and older survivors have been significantly less likely to seek help, especially from IPV shelters in addition to those reasons already mention (Cho et al, 2020). Conventional strategies intended to empower survivors in re-establishing safety and self-determination following a violent incident or in the context of an abusive relationship can miscomprehend the lived realities of trans older people, as for example when a trans individual may have experienced a systemic lack of love and care, and one of the only people that loves and cares for them is also abusive and the level of isolation experienced (Jordan et al, 2020). There is also some debate about the use of the term 'hate crime' to describe what is more complex for people with diverse gender identities (Carr et al, 2019). Relationships with and support from community-based organisations supporting LGBT+ are not straightforward, as Jordan et al's (2020) participants identified a fear of being tokenised or overburdening LGBT+ services, or the possibility of being referred to such services without their consent. Overall, the evidence suggests that trans people do not on the whole access DA specialist services and social care provision. This inevitably leads to greater reliance on self-care and friendship families (Donovan and Barnes, 2020) such as counsellors or therapists with the danger that DA is understood as personal relationship 'troubles' resulting from personal failings and reinforcing low expectations of mainstream providers (Donovan and Hester, 2015).

Influencing and shaping practice in DA

So, what can practitioners do to make a step-up change to support trans people experiencing DA in later life given the insufficient research and practice evidence on their experiences? One unique project in the United States called FORGE has addressed this intersection of trans violence and ageing and talks about the 'small-t' traumas (typically labelled minority stress and micro-aggressions, such as ongoing insults), as well as the more commonly recognised 'large-T' traumas (sexual assault, hate crimes and DA). Research suggests that there is a re-emergence of trauma in later life, the symptoms of which become worse as a survivor ages (Munson, 2016). However, as we have seen, trans older people do not have access to support and can become trapped in an abusive relationship. FORGE has responded to the lack of training or lack of information on trans issues or the after-effects of trauma or violence on trans people by addressing these gaps. Trauma-informed services made relevant to trans communities is one example of good practice that practitioners can draw from.

More work is needed detailing trans people's experiences that accounts for the intersections between older age and other sources of inequality/minoritised status. There is value in employing an intersectionality framework for scrutinising trans people's narratives of abuse and maltreatment. This serves as a reminder that lived experiences are often correlated with multiple, not singular, aspects of a person's identity and social location (Rogers, 2021). Practice tools are needed to capture the full range of IPV experiences impacting trans older people, to develop gender-sensitive IPV screening and provide affirmative interventions including counselling practices. These need to address the syndemic effects of IPV (meaning that these include both social marginalisation *and* health outcomes such as substance use and mental health) (King et al, 2021). In the UK, the charity SaveLives (nd) has developed a risk checklist called DASH (see Table 9.1), which has been developed to support identification when DA, 'honour'-based violence and/or stalking are disclosed. DASH offers additional questions to enable practitioners to identify specific risks in DA situations where the victim/survivor identifies as LGBTQ+, with two specific questions tailored to trans and/or non-binary victims/survivors which are outlined in Table 9.1.

In addressing one practical challenge, Cook-Daniels (2015) suggests the preparation or provision of 'get away kits' which contain necessary medical and legal documentation required for trans survivors to establish their identity (particularly for individuals in transition), medications and devices (such as hormones, binders, dilators and so on) that may be required should they need to leave home quickly. As some trans people may find it difficult to locate clothing in their size and preferred gender, these kits should also include numerous pieces of clothing in appropriate sizes. However, this may not be practical for a lot of older trans people with disabilities, chronic health conditions, limited mobility or dependency on others, where the idea of 'getting away' will not be feasible and whose choices will be even further limited if they need to leave home or enter institutional care as an alternative.

Table 9.1: SafeLives DASH LGBTQ+ questions

SafeLives DASH LGBTQ+ questions				
	Yes	No	n/k	Comments
1 Does (...) blame the abuse on your LGBTQ+ identity?				
2 Are you out to your family, friends, wider support network? If No, has (...) threatened to out you or have they outed you to family, work, children, friends, education, services, religious or other communities? If No, has (...) threatened that no one else will support you or respect your identity?				
3 Is this your first relationship since identifying as an LGB and/or T person?				
4 As an LGBTQ+ person, do you fear or have you experienced 'honour based' violence or forced marriage as a result of your family's/religion's/culture's/communities' beliefs regarding sexuality/gender identity? If Yes, has (...) threatened you with being taken out of the country?				
5 Have you ever experienced or been threatened with 'so-called' conversion therapies (this may include but is not limited to being prayed for, being beaten or made to ingest something, exorcisms, corrective rape) If Yes, was this in the past six months? Or over six months ago?				

Trans- and non-binary-specific questions – to be asked in addition to the previous questions if the service user identifies as trans and/or non-binary

	Yes	No	n/k	Comments
1 Does (...) try to prevent you from expressing your gender identity, refuse to use your pronouns and/or deadname you?				
2 Does (...) try to prevent you from accessing transition-related healthcare (for example hormones, speech therapy, surgery)?				

Source: SafeLives. A pdf version can be freely downloaded from https://safelives.org.uk/sites/default/files/resources/Dash%20without%20guidance.pdf

Summary learning points

The following key points for prevention and intervention can be referred to by practitioners and services when working with trans people experiencing DA and IPV in later life.

Prevention

- Recognise and address power dynamics when working with people in difficult relationships in which one partner is trans (King et al, 2021).
- Support trans survivors by focusing on person-centred practice and approaches which position trans people as 'experts' of their experiences with control over decision making (Rogers, 2016). This is significant for older people with care and support needs, whose autonomy may be constricted and/or removed by others including within care settings.
- Review and develop IPV-screening practices that address the intersection of ageing and trans issues and use an intersectional lens and a life course/narrative approach (Ghandour et al, 2015).
- Address and act to promote gender neutrality of IPV services (Rogers, 2021).
- Ensure that any safety planning recognises barriers for older people in the tailoring of care and support for DA.
- Give attention to expanding older trans persons' (sometimes limited) social networks which build capacity for more options in disclosing/escaping IPV.
- Keep up to date with research and evidence to inform best practice with trans older people to help address the gaps they face.

Intervention

- Commission services from community-based organisations to provide specialist support for DA/IPV for older trans people.
- Address the limitations of single-sex spaces in mainstream support.
- Support and resource peer-support groups developed by and for trans people and their communities, which will facilitate recognition, advocacy and support for IPV/DA and impacted areas of health and wellbeing (Jordan et al, 2020).
- Allocate resources to train care professionals in IPV/DA that are co-produced with trans older people.
- Inform professionals, practitioners and providers of gender-affirming services which recognise the long-term benefits of transition. These prevent IPV/DA and promote improved quality of life, greater relationship satisfaction, higher self-esteem and confidence (Cornell University, 2018).

- Develop education and outreach campaigns on trans ageing IPV/DV as a public health priority which addresses the intersecting nature of discrimination and victimisation. Involve multidisciplinary services and community organisations to champion trans ageing needs (Saad et al, 2020).
- Map the community resources available for trans people in later life in your local area and include these in induction and team work to support those experiencing IPV and DA (Willis et al, 2022).
- Conduct local research on trans people's experiences of IPV and DA and/or disaggregate existing data on protected characteristics (gender and sexual identities, age, ethnicity, disability and so on) to provide insights into older trans people's experiences and needs.

Finally, researchers, service providers and community members need to collaborate to research this knowledge gap and the wider problem of discrimination and violence against trans persons. This could contribute to the development of trans-positive, evidence-based models of practice grounded in the experiences of trans people in later life.

Note

[1] 'Passing' is an expression related to the social evaluation on whether a trans person's gender is perceived as deviant or not, attributing validity to it (see Duque, 2017). The term is however controversial and debated since that alignment, defined by social norms and expectations, may be related to an attempt by trans people to fit into heterocisnormative and binary standards.

References

AEA v EHRC (2021) EWHC 1623 (Admin) Case no: CO/4116/2020 HTML version of judgment approved. Held at Royal Courts of Justice Strand, London, on Thursday, 6 May 2021. London: Crown Copyright, Available from: https://oldsquare.co.uk/wp-content/uploads/2021/11/R-on-application-of-AEA-v-EHRC-2021-EWHC-1623-Admin.pdf

Arayasirikul, S., Turner, C., Trujillo, D. Sicro, S.L., Scheer, S., McFarland, W. et al (2022) 'A global cautionary tale: discrimination and violence against trans women worsen despite investments in public resources and improvements in health insurance access and utilization of health care', *International Journal of Equity and Health*, 21: 32, Available from: https://doi.org/10.1186/s12939-022-01632-5

Beaulaurier, R.L., Seff, L.R., Newman, F.L. and Dunlop, B. (2005) 'Internal barriers to help seeking for middle-aged and older women who experience intimate partner violence', *Journal of Elder Abuse & Neglect*, 17(3): 53–74.

Bornstein, D.R., Fawcett, J., Sullivan, M., Senturia, K.D. and Shiu-Thornton, S. (2006) 'Understanding the experiences of lesbian, bisexual and trans survivors of domestic violence: a qualitative study', *Journal of Homosexuality*, 51(1): 159–81.

Breiding, M.J. and Armour, B.S. (2015) 'The association between disability and intimate partner violence in the United States', *Annals of Epidemiology*, 25(6): 455–7.

Brown, N.T. and Herman, J.L. (2015) 'Intimate partner violence and sexual abuse among LGBT people: a review of existing research', Williams Institute, UCLA School of Law, Available from: https://williamsinstitute.law.ucla.edu/publications/ipv-sex-abuse-lgbt-people/

Carr, S., Hafford-Letchfield, T., Faulkner, A., Megele, C., Gould, D., Khisa, C. et al (2019) 'Keeping control: a user-led exploratory study of mental health service user experiences of targeted violence and abuse in the context of adult safeguarding in England', *Health and Social Care in the Community*, 27(5): 781–92.

Cook-Daniels, L. (2015) 'Intimate partner violence in transgender couples: "power and control" in a specific cultural context', *Partner Abuse*, 6(1): 126–39.

Cook-Daniels, L. and Munson, M. (2010) 'Sexual violence, elder abuse, and sexuality of transgender adults, age 50+: results of three surveys', *Journal of GLBT Family Studies*, 6(2): 142–77.

Cornell University (2018) 'What does the scholarly research say about the effect of gender transition on transgender well-being?' [online literature review], Available from: https://whatweknow.inequality.cornell.edu/topics/lgbt-equality/what-does-the-scholarly-research-say-about-the-well-being-of-transgender-people/

Dong, X., Simon, M., Mendes de Leon, C., Fulmer, T., Beck, T., Hebert, L. et al (2009) 'Elder self-neglect and abuse and mortality risk in a community-dwelling population', *Journal of the American Medical Association*, 302(5): 517–26.

Donovan, C. and Barnes, R. (2020) 'Help-seeking among lesbian, gay, bisexual and/or transgender victims/survivors of domestic violence and abuse: the impacts of cisgendered heteronormativity and invisibility', *Journal of Sociology*, 56(4): 554–70.

Donovan, C. and Hester, M. (2015) *Domestic Violence and Sexuality: What's Love Got to Do with It?*, Bristol: Bristol University Press.

Duque, T. (2017) '"We always have courage": identification, recognition and experiences of (not) passing by man and/or woman', *Cadernos Pagu*, 51. Published by Universidade Estadual de Campinas, Brazil

Equality and Human Rights Commission (2022) 'Separate and single-sex service providers: a guide on the Equality Act sex and gender reassignment provisions; guidance', Available from: https://www.equalityhumanrights.com/sites/default/files/guidance-separate-and-single-sex-service-providers-equality-act-sex-and-gender-reassignment-exceptions.pdf

Flentje, A., Leon, A., Carrico, A., Zheng, D. and Dilley, J. (2016) 'Mental and physical health among homeless sexual and gender minorities in a major urban US city', *Journal of Urban Health: Bulletin of the New York Academy of Medicine*, 93(6): 997–1009.

FORGE (2005) 'Sexual violence in the transgender community survey, unpublished data', Available from: https://forge-forward.org/resources/anti-violence/

Gelles, R.J. (1997) *Intimate Violence in Families* (3rd edn), London: Sage Publications.

Goffman, E. (1979 [1963]) *Stigma: Notes on the Management of Spoiled Identity*, Harmondsworth: Penguin Books

Grant, J.M, Mottet, L.A., Tanis, J., Harrison, J., Herman, J. and Mara, K. (2011) 'Injustice at every turn: a report of the National Transgender Discrimination Survey', Washington, DC: National Center for Transgender Equality and National Gay and Lesbian Task Force.

Guadalupe-Diaz, X.L. and Jasinski, J. (2017) '"I wasn't a priority, I wasn't a victim": challenges in help seeking for transgender survivors of intimate partner violence', *Violence Against Women*, 23(6): 772–92.

Hawkey, A.J., Ussher, J.M., Liamputtong, P., Brahmaputra, M., Sekar, J.A., Perz, J. et al (2021) 'Trans women's responses to sexual violence: vigilance, resilience, and need for support', *Archives of Sexual Behavior*, 50(7): 3201–22.

Hillman, J. (2020) 'Intimate partner violence among older LGBT adults: unique risk factors, issues in reporting and treatment, and recommendations for research, practice, and policy', in B. Russell (ed) *Gender and Intimate Partner Violence*, Cham: Springer, pp 237–54.

Hillman, J. (2022) 'Lifetime prevalence of intimate partner violence and health-related outcomes among transgender adults aged 50 and older', *Gerontologist*, 9(62/2): 212–22.

Home Office (2018) 'Domestic violence and abuse: new definition', Available from: https://www.gov.uk/guidance/domestic-violence-and-abuse

James, S.E., Herman, J.L., Rankin, S., Keisling, M., Mottet, L. and Anafi, M. (2016) 'The report of the 2015 U.S. transgender survey: National Center for Transgender Equality', Available from: https://www.ustranssurvey.org

Jauk, D. (2013) 'Gender violence revisited: Lessons from violent victimization of transgender identified individuals', *Sexualities*, 16(7): 807–25.

Johns, M.M., Lowry, R., Rasberry, C.N., Dunville, R., Robin, L., Pampati, S. et al (2018) 'Violence victimization, substance use and suicide risk among sexual minority high school students: United States, 2015–2017', *Morbidity and Mortality Weekly Report*, 67(43): 1211–15.

Jordan, S.P., Mehrotra, G.R. and Fujikawa, K.A. (2020) 'Mandating inclusion: critical trans perspectives on domestic and sexual violence advocacy', *Violence Against Women*, 26(6–7): 531–54.

King, W.M., Restar, A. and Operario, D. (2021) 'Exploring multiple forms of intimate partner violence in a gender and racially/ethnically diverse sample of transgender adults', *Journal of Interpersonal Violence*, 36(19–20): 10477–98.

Langenderfer-Magruder, L., Whitfield, D.L., Walls, N.E., Kattari, S.K and Ramos, D. (2016) 'Experiences of intimate partner violence and subsequent police reporting among lesbian, gay, bisexual, transgender, and queer adults in Colorado: comparing rates of cisgender and transgender victimization', *Journal of Interpersonal Violence*, 31(5): 855–71.

Magić, J. and Kelley, P. (2018) 'LGBT+ people's experiences of domestic abuse: a report on Galop's domestic abuse advocacy service', London: Galop, the LGBT+ anti-violence charity.

Messinger, A.M., Guadalupe-Diaz, X.L. and Kurdyla, V. (2022) 'Transgender polyvictimization in the U.S. transgender survey', *Journal of Interpersonal Violence*, 37(19–20): 18810–36.

Munson, M. (2016) 'FORGE's trauma-informed trans aging work', *Generations: Journal of the American Society on Aging*, 40(20): 71–2.

Namaste, V.E. (2000) *Invisible Lives: The Erasure of Transsexual and Transgendered People*. Chicago, London: University of Chicago Press.

Parry, M.N. and O'Neal, E.N. (2015) 'Help-seeking behavior among same-sex intimate partner violence victims: an intersectional argument', *Criminology*, 16(1): 51–67.

Pearce, R., Erikainen, S. and Vincent, B. (2020) 'TERF wars: an introduction', *The Sociological Review*, 68(4): 677–98.

Peixoto, E.M., de Azevedo Oliveira Knupp, V.M., Soares, J.R.T., Depret, D.G., de Oliveira Souza, C., Messina, M.E.D. et al (2022) 'Interpersonal violence and passing: results from a Brazilian trans-specific cross-sectional study', *Journal of Interpersonal Violence*, 37(15–16): 14397–410.

Rogers, M. (2016) 'Breaking down barriers: exploring the potential for social care practice with trans survivors of domestic abuse', *Health and Social Care in the Community*, 24(1): 68–76.

Rogers, M. (2017) 'Transphobic "honour"-based abuse: a conceptual tool', *Sociology*, 51(2): 225–40.

Rogers, M.M. (2021) 'Exploring the domestic abuse narratives of trans and nonbinary people and the role of cisgenderism in identity abuse, misgendering, and pathologizing', *Violence Against Women*, 27(12–13): 2187–207.

Saad, M., Burley, J.F., Miljanovski, M., Macdonald, S., Bradley, C. and Du Mont, J. (2020) 'Planning an intersectoral network of healthcare and community leaders to advance trans-affirming care for sexual assault survivors', *Healthcare Management Forum*, 33(2): 65–9.

Safe Lives (nd) Resources for identifying the risk victims face, https://safelives.org.uk/practice-support/resources-identifying-risk-victims-face

Schilt, K. and Wiswall, M. (2008) 'Before and after: gender transitions, human capital, and workplace experiences', *The B.E. Journal of Economic Analysis & Policy*, 8(1): 1–28.

Schultz, J.W. (2020) 'Supporting transmasculine survivors of sexual assault and intimate partner violence: reflections from peer support facilitation', *Sociological Inquiry*, 90(2): 293–315.

Scottish Transgender Alliance (2011) 'Out of sight, out of mind? Transgender people's experiences of domestic abuse', Available from: file:///C:/Users/kxb19198/Downloads/trans_domestic_abuse.pdf

Seelman, K.L., Colón-Diaz, M.J.P., LeCroix, R.H., Xavier-Brier, M. and Kattari, L. (2017) 'Transgender non-inclusive healthcare and delaying care because of fear: connections to general health and mental health among transgender adults', *Transgender Health*, 2(1): 17–28.

Serano, J. (2007) *Whipping Girl: A Transsexual Woman on Sexism and the Scapegoating of Femininity*. Seal Press.

Silva, I.C.B, Araújo, E.C., Santana, A.D.S, Moura, J.W.S, Ramalho, M.N.A and Abreu, P.D. (2022) 'Gender violence perpetrated against trans women', *Revista Brasileira de Enfermagem*, 75(suppl 2): e20210173.

Smith, L.R., Yore, J., Triplett, D.P., Urada, L., Nemoto, T. and Raj, A. (2017) 'Impact of sexual violence across the lifespan on HIV risk behaviors among transgender women and cisgender people living with HIV', *Journal of Acquired Immune Deficiency Syndrome*, 75(4): 408–16.

Sterzing, P.R., Gartner, R.E., Goldbach, J.T., McGeough, B.L., Ratliff, G.A. and Johnson, K.C. (2019) 'Polyvictimization prevalence rates for sexual and gender minority adolescents: breaking down the silos of victimization research', *Psychology of Violence*, 9(4): 419–30.

Stotzer, R.L. (2009) 'Violence against transgender people: a review of United States data', *Aggression and Violent Behavior*, 14(3): 170–9.

Swan, L.E.T, Henry, R.S, Smith, E.R., Aguayo Arelis, A., Rabago Barajas, B.V. and Perrin, P.B. (2021) 'Discrimination and intimate partner violence victimization and perpetration among a convenience sample of LGBT individuals in Latin America', *Journal of Interpersonal Violence*, 36(15–16): 8520–37.

Talusan, M. (2016) 'Unerased: counting transgender lives', Mic Network, Available from: https://mic.com/unerased/

Taylor, N., Fraser, H. and Riggs, D.W. (2016) 'Domestic violence and companion animals in the context of LGBT people's relationships', *Sexualities*, 22(5–6): 821–36.

Trans Murder Monitoring Global Update (2023) Available from: https://transrespect.org/en/trans-murder-monitoring-2023/

UK Government (2010) Equality Act. Available from: https://www.legislation.gov.uk/ukpga/2010/15/contents

Valentine, S.E., Peitzmeier, S.M., King, D.S., O'Cleirigh, C., Marquez, S.M., Presley, C. et al (2017) 'Disparities in exposure to intimate partner violence among transgender/gender nonconforming and sexual minority primary care patients', *LGBT Health*, 4(4): 260–7.

Warmling, D., Lindner, S.R. and Coelho, E.B.S. (2017) 'Intimate partner violence prevalence in the elderly and associated factors: systematic review', *Ciencia & Saude Coletiva*, 22(9): 3111–25.

Waters, E. and Yacka-Bible, S. (2017) 'A crisis of hate: a mid year report on lesbian, gay, bisexual, transgender and queer hate violence homicides', National Coalition of Anti-Violence Programs, Available from: https://avp.org/wp-content/uploads/2017/08/NCAVP-A-Crisisof-Hate-Final.pdf

Westwood, S. (2019) 'Abuse and older lesbian, gay bisexual, and trans (LGBT) people: a commentary and research agenda', *Journal of Elder Abuse & Neglect*, 31(2): 97–114.

Willis, P., Toze, M. and Hafford-Letchfield, T. (2022) 'Working with older trans people: practice tool', Dartington: Research in Practice for Adults, Available from: https://www.researchinpractice.org.uk/adults/publications/2022/november/working-with-older-trans-people-practice-tool-2022/

Willis, P., Raithby, M., Dobbs, C., Evans, E. and Bishop, J. (2021) '"I'm going to live my life for me": trans ageing, care, and older trans and gender non-conforming adults' expectations of and concerns for later life', *Ageing & Society*, 41(12): 2792–813.

Witten, T.M. (2014) 'End of life, chronic illness, and trans-identities', *Journal of Social Work in End-of-Life & Palliative Care*, 10(1): 34–58.

World Health Organization (nd) 'Intimate partner violence', Available from: https://apps.who.int/violence-info/intimate-partner-violence

Zanghellini, A. (2020) 'Philosophical problems with the gender-critical feminist argument against trans inclusion', *SAGE Open*, 10(2), Available from: https://doi.org/10.1177/2158244020927029

Over to you

This section provides three suggested learning activities for readers that connect explicitly with the content and themes that have arisen in the seven chapters in Part II. These critically examine the practices, views and attitudes of healthcare and social welfare professionals towards older trans people and have a focus on taking responsibility for education and professional development that support access to supportive and inclusive services.

Practitioners can use these learning activities to help develop and share knowledge, skills and values that will inform the development of affirmative and person-centred support for older trans people by:

- extending your own personal and professional knowledge through relevant desktop research or practitioner enquiry;
- facilitating critical reflection and learning through active discussion in your team and service.

Educators and trainers can use these activities:

- to include trans ageing issues in the education and training of the workforce;
- to guide the aim and focus of trans issues drawing on the relevant evidence provided.

Managers can use these activities to:

- embed the relevant topics, areas and learning resources into the recruitment, induction, supervision, appraisal and staff career progression process;
- keep a record of key activities that can be drawn upon in practice reviews or benchmarks to demonstrate how the needs of older trans people are being addressed, including the potential to demonstrate legal compliance during statutory regulatory activities.

Activity 3: The use of self and literacy on gender and sexual identities

Being open and accessible in how you communicate affirmation for gender diverse people in later life requires willingness and confidence in enabling individuals and their loved ones in the expression of their identities and relationships.

This reflective activity aims to promote your own awareness and insights into gender and sexual identities in later life and to identify the barriers to establishing rapport.

It draws on the social GGRRAAACCEEESSS model (Gender Geography Race Religion Age Ability Appearance Culture Class/Caste Education Employment Ethnicity Spirituality Sexuality Sexual orientation) (Burnham, 2012) which helps practitioners to recognise factors which affect our position, powers and privileges. These factors influence relationships and interactions with others and can be used to deconstruct the power relationship between a practitioner and the older person when exploring the relevance and meaning of sexuality, sexual and gender identities, and what the practitioner or professional might bring to these interactions.

- Which of the social GGRRAAACCEEESSS factors have most influenced your own experience of gender and sexual identity, and how might this shape your professional practice in this area?

Factors	Your experience
Gender	
Geography	
Race	
Religion	
Age	
Ability	
Appearance	
Culture	
Class/caste	
Education	

- How do visible, invisible, voiced and unvoiced experiences of these factors affect your understanding and expectations about expression of gender and sexuality in later life?
- How do visible, invisible and unvoiced experience of these factors affect your understanding and expectations about older people's expression of gender and sexuality?
- What training have you received to enable your role of supporting gender diverse people in later life?
- What extra training or learning would benefit your work with this population, and who/how could this be best provided?

- What other sources of support, advice and guidance in your place of work could be tapped into to meet your learning needs in this area?

Activity 4: On the spot: preparing for anti-discriminatory and affirmative practice

The following scenarios can be used by individuals or teams to facilitate discussion about how to respond to transphobia and discrimination and to provide support for gender diverse older people in different settings.

1. Your administrative colleague Mindy is telling you about their weekend while taking a coffee break at work and casually mentions that a 'trannie' has moved in next door to his brother which they were laughing about.
2. You refer Uri, a 74-year-old trans man, to his family doctor to talk about his options for affirmative gender support, and Uri reports back to you that the doctor told him that given the long waiting list for the regional gender clinic that 'it wasn't worth him going down that road at his age'.
3. When supporting Abi, who is non-binary and wants to consider supported living, the provider tells you that it's going to be hard for Abi to fit in with the other residents, and if they move in, they should be advised to "keep a low profile".
4. During an assessment in the local hospital with Margaret to consider her care needs after discharge, the nurse reports that Margaret has been difficult and aggressive to other residents and given her strong physique may be a threat to other women on the ward.

Learning how to practise in an anti-discriminatory or culturally competent way requires a basic understanding of discrimination from its basis in cognitive or learned processes through to the active formation of prejudices and how this informs oppression. Having discussed these scenarios, try to articulate the ethical and legal basis of your anti-discriminatory practice, including identifying any professional requirements that you are aligned to such as your professional code of practice and the guiding legislation. Further, give attention to a form of words that you could practise and use in more effectively responding to the protagonist in these scenarios in a way that conveys your commitment and offers to educate rather than to silence or be 'politically correct' for its own sake.

Activity 5: Continuously improving your own knowledge, skills and commitment to trans inclusion

Being a trans ally or trans activist requires us to constantly listen and learn as well as questioning and unlearning ideas that we may have been brought up with so that we can be open to new ways of understanding gender in society. The following activities are suggested as a means of making a step-up improvement as well as maintaining your commitment to trans inclusion.

Learning activities	Suggested actions
Keeping up to date with research and practice evidence on trans issues.	Set up 'update' alerts with relevant publications. Visit the websites of local organisations who are trans affirmative or trans led and download any research reports. Invite researchers to share their research/practice findings via a team webinar. Discuss your reading with a colleague and record learning in your record of continuing professional development.
Arrange a dedicated learning event in your team or service.	Consider how you can involve trans people in the design and delivery of learning events and in producing learning materials. Request relevant learning materials and events and material from your Learning and Development team to address knowledge gaps.
Establish a formal mechanism in your work for discussing trans inclusion regularly.	Put trans issues on your team meeting agenda and offer to lead a discussion. Request a meeting with senior leaders, HR and trade unions to discuss what the service and organisation is doing to promote trans rights.
Taking up the role of trans ally or champion.	Look for opportunities to undertake additional learning and development to become a named person for trans colleagues and people who use services to contact directly.
Critical reflection on your practice with trans people in later life.	Introduce your learning needs and experiences to forums such as supervision and annual reviews and establish some objectives for your learning and development. Use critical reflective tools to review and evaluate your practice in this area.

Reference

Burnham, J. (2012) 'Developments in the social GGRRAAACCEEESSS: visible–invisible and voiced/unvoiced', in I. Krause (ed) *Culture and Reflexivity in Systemic Psychotherapy: Mutual Perspectives*, London: Karnac, pp 139–60.

PART III

Making care practices more inclusive: perspectives on improving care and support for trans people in later life

10

Trans history as cultural competence

Kit Heyam

Introduction

Contemporary anti-trans political discourse has rendered knowledge of trans history inextricable from trans allyship. Leveraging the idea of trans people's newness – sometimes as a trend which can be trivially dismissed, sometimes as an emergent threat against which new laws must be forged to protect the gender-conforming majority – anti-trans campaigners have politicised the very idea of trans historicity (Heyam, 2022). While it is certainly true that a combination of increased trans visibility and (increasingly fragile) advances in legal equality has resulted in increased numbers coming out as trans and seeking medical transition, the long, global history of non-conforming and de-essentialised conceptualisations of gender is also increasingly well documented (Feinberg, 1994; Stryker, 2017; Raskolnikov et al, 2021; Heyam, 2022). As a result, the ethical and political importance of knowing and talking about the existence of trans history is also increasingly well understood among trans-supportive individuals.

Yet for practitioners working with older trans adults, knowledge of trans history is not simply valuable as part of a generalised ethical commitment to equality and allyship. At a deeper, more systemic level, I want to argue here that knowledge of trans history is an undervalued form of cultural competence in supporting older trans people. As such, it deserves to be understood as an integral part of professional development for practitioners in this area: neither situated as primarily a tactic for combatting anti-trans political arguments, nor confined to focal points such as LGBT+ History Month, but acknowledged as a central element of professional practice.

In framing knowledge of trans history as 'cultural competence', I want to align it with other kinds of knowledge necessary for effective, empathetic care: to emphasise that it is of equal value to knowledge of service users' cultural or religious values and practices and their often culturally specific understandings of themselves and their place in their communities. A lack of cultural competence can lead practitioners to make inaccurate assumptions about those they support, leading to the provision of care that fails to meet their needs. By contrast, developing cultural competence can facilitate person-centred support and build effective relationships between practitioners and those they care for.

In the first part of this short chapter, I argue that the desire to be 'up to date' in concepts and terminology of trans experience does not always effectively prepare practitioners to support older trans people. I provide a historical overview of changes in the terminology used to describe trans and gender-non-conforming experience since the 19th century, followed by an outline of how understandings of what it means to be trans have concurrently shifted: the move away from a medical model of transness that conflated it with intersex embodiment, the shift from an emphasis on privacy and 'stealth' life to one on openness and pride, and the changing relationship between gender and sexuality. I also explore the experiences of those who transitioned, medically and/or socially, in the 1960s and 1970s, and show how this might affect those people's decision making and relationships with medical professionals today.

In the second part, I argue that a deeper understanding of trans history can help us to think more critically about how we validate trans identities and self-articulations. What *feels* like a real trans identity to us – one we should believe, take seriously, and treat with respect – and what doesn't? The structures which shape these processes of validation or invalidation are not self-evident: as I show, they were produced by the specific contexts of the mid-20th-century gender clinic. Understanding the factors that forged our contemporary ideas of what makes someone 'really trans' is, I argue, essential to recognising how they may limit our capacity to treat all trans people with respect and care.

While my analysis here focuses on Western understandings of trans experience – indeed, I would argue that the use of the word 'trans' to describe non-Western gendered experiences should be approached with caution (Heyam, 2022) – my central contention about the value of historical understanding for ethical, person-centred work with older people is transcultural. Practitioners working in non-Western contexts would, I suggest, benefit from applying a similar approach.

"I want to make sure I'm up to date": changing terminology, concepts and experiences

When I deliver trans awareness training to any group, from university staff to caring professionals, I ask attendees what has brought them to a session. Among the variety of responses which follow, a persistent thread emerges: attendees are especially afraid of being 'out of date'. "I just need an update on what the right terminology is now", they tell me. "Everything's changing so fast – I want to make sure I'm up to date." "My teenager knows way more about this stuff than me!"

Certainly, respectful treatment of trans people from a contemporary perspective is an essential part of such training. Moreover, it has been shown to be especially crucial for practitioners working with older trans adults, who are more likely to experience specific challenges, from harassment to bathroom access (Bailey, 2012, p 64; Fabbre, 2015, p 145; Porter et al, 2016; Pearce, 2018). But alongside the introduction of my training attendees to the current most dominant terms, it feels crucial for me to emphasise that self-definition remains paramount. Knowing basic umbrella terms is useful in equipping attendees to work respectfully with trans people but arguably not as useful as giving individuals the opportunity to self-describe on their *own* terms – even if such self-descriptions are at odds with those of others. Indeed, as Marta V. Vicente has cogently argued, umbrella terms like 'transgender' can threaten to '[render] invisible all the nuances and multiple identities of trans★ people' (Vicente, 2021, pp 436–7).

Prioritising a principle of self-definition avoids the imposition of an inadequate terminological or conceptual framework on to individuals who have not chosen it. In this way, it can be usefully understood as a form of cultural competence, analogous to the need to avoid the (often colonial) imposition of Western terms and concepts on to other cultures for which they are unfit. In fact, the analogy is particularly apt with regard to gender: not only are White and/or Western trans people liable to impose Western gender hierarchies and binaries on to non-Western cultures, thereby misrepresenting and tokenising those cultures' often more complex gender-non-conforming experiences (Porter et al, 2016, pp 378–9; Heyam, 2022), but the homogenisation of the term 'transgender' can be seen as a form of 'gender purity' with oppressive political roots, having 'historically developed in tandem with racial purity' (Vicente, 2021, pp 437–8).

In light of these diverse understandings of gender and these problems with conceptual homogenisation, practitioners working with older trans adults should be concerned not merely with 'up-to-date' terminology but with the fact that older trans people may understand and articulate their identities differently from the younger people whose experiences are often centred in general-purpose trans awareness training. Clearly, older trans people are a diverse demographic – not merely culturally and socioeconomically but also in terms of how recently they began different aspects of their transition, or their age in 'trans time' (Pearce, 2018). The terminology and concepts of gender used by chronologically older trans people who transitioned recently, and the experiences of those people, may well have more in common with those of chronologically younger trans people than with those of their chronological peers who transitioned longer ago. Yet the force of 'trans time' is not absolute: any chronologically older trans person, regardless of when they transitioned, has lived through more cultural changes relating to gender than a chronologically younger trans person, and this may well have shaped their self-understanding over time. This is likely intensified by the fact that many chronologically older trans people consider or plan their transitions over long periods (Fabbre, 2014, p 9).

The historical narratives outlined in this chapter are in no way intended to homogenise older trans people as a conservative group who are likely to reject outright 21st-century forms of self-description and self-understanding. Instead, they proceed from the standpoint that trans-aware practitioners in all fields can develop their practice in a more ethical direction by being more fully prepared for the diversity of self-understanding that might exist among their trans stakeholders; and that among older trans people, such preparation may benefit from historical understanding alongside other forms of knowledge.

Naming trans experience

Since the late 19th century, Western terminology for what might broadly be understood as trans experience has exploded in diversity and complexity. German sexologist Magnus Hirschfeld popularised the term 'transvestite' to refer specifically to those who identified and/or presented in ways different from their sex assigned at birth in his 1910 book *Die Transvestiten* (The transvestites). Unhappy with the emphasis 'transvestite' placed on dress over identity, Hirschfeld was the first to refer to 'psychic transsexualism' in 1923; this term was first used in English by David O. Cauldwell and popularised by the American sexologist Harry Benjamin (Ekins and King, 2001; Siotos et al, 2019, p 132). 'Transsexual' became, for several decades, the dominant term to describe people living as a gender different from the one they were assigned at birth, but it did not replace 'transvestite'; instead, the two coexisted, often spoken of as two aspects of one community (Burns, 2018a, p 26). Subsequently, during the 1970s, the term 'transgender' emerged among gender-non-conforming communities – initially as a semantic alternative to 'transsexual' (indicating that an individual lived as a gender different from the one they were assigned at birth but had not 'changed their sex' through medical transition) – but later, and increasingly from the 1990s onwards, as a political alternative which rejected the idea that trans people should be defined primarily through their bodily characteristics and sought to draw connections between all gender-non-conforming people rather than entrenching divisions based on medical history (Vicente, 2021, p 430). More recently, the dominance of 'transgender' as an umbrella term has led trans communities to narrow its scope, excluding once again those who *dress* but do not *identify* in ways distinct from their assigned gender and who might use terms such as 'gender-non-conforming', as well as the older term 'transvestite', to describe themselves (Vicente, 2021, p 430; Heyam, 2022, pp 96–100). Concurrently, some trans people now seek to reclaim the term 'transsexual', whether to emphasise their solidarity with the history of trans activism or to highlight the specific experiences of those who undertake medical transition.

This brief overview demonstrates the rapidity with which terminology and definitions have shifted over the past 150 years. Someone who transitioned medically in the 1960s might at the time have described themself as 'transsexual'; someone who went through the same process 50 years later might reject that term. Someone who began their transition in the 1970s might feel comfortable with the term 'transvestite' and excluded by 21st-century trans communities' frequent rejection of it; someone who transitioned in the 2000s might find that term sensationalised and outdated. Even those who transitioned around the same time as each other might, of course, have accessed different kinds of community support and thus come to understand themselves through a different terminological lens. The danger of presentist trans awareness training which dismisses terms like 'transsexual' and 'transvestite' as offensive and outdated, then, is that it may render practitioners working with older trans people less able to accept and respect their self-descriptions at face value.

Conceptualising trans experience

This is not, moreover, a simple matter of 'different words for the same thing'. On the contrary, the very concept of what it means to be trans has shifted over the same historical period with similar dynamism. Mid-20th-century biomedical understanding often conflated trans identity with intersex embodiment (Gill-Peterson, 2018, pp 16–17, 60, 80, 141; Griffiths, 2018), and this was reflected in trans people's own self-understanding (Amin, 2018; Gill-Peterson, 2018, pp 16, 80; Griffiths, 2018). Combined with an emphasis in trans medicine on the desire for medical transition as an essential criterion for a diagnosis of transsexualism (later gender dysphoria) (Velocci, 2021, p 474), this biological conceptualisation of trans experience is more likely to result in an understanding of transness as primarily a medical condition to be fixed through hormones and/or surgery rather than an identity category. In our contemporary political context, where (in spite of increasing anti-trans hostility) trans people often celebrate being trans as a difference to be proud of and see a focus on medical transition as invasive, practitioners working with older trans people should be prepared to find different attitudes among this group.

Concurrently, before around the 1990s, those transitioning faced what we might term a 'stealth imperative': they were heavily encouraged, sometimes required, by clinicians to treat their transition as the start of a new life, cutting ties with old friends and workplaces and concealing their trans status from everyone around them (Catherwood, 2015, p 49; Porter et al, 2016, p 370;

Burns, 2018a, p 31; Pearce, 2018). Even those chronologically older trans people who transitioned recently, and were therefore not directly subject to this stealth imperative, may have internalised the ideas and values behind it; indeed, this may have directly shaped their decisions to wait before transitioning. When combined with more biological and medicalised understandings of trans experience, this may result in some older trans people feeling less inclined to disclose, talk about or express pride in their trans status, and/or feeling less kinship with those who do.

The 20th-century conceptual overlap between trans experience and intersex embodiment was mirrored by a similar, but often more contested, conceptual overlap between gender and sexuality – specifically, between what we would now call trans experience and gay/lesbian experience. The late-19th and early 20th-century sexological concept of 'inversion' codified the idea that attraction to the same sex as one was assigned at birth was the product of psychological gender inversion: if a person assigned male at birth (AMAB) was attracted to men, that was because they were psychologically female. These understandings were carried forward into mid-20th-century understandings of trans experience, including criteria for medical transition, and were again reflected in the way some trans people described themselves (Gill-Peterson, 2018, pp 142, 60). For clinicians in much of the 20th century, an essential criterion for medical transition was that a trans person be attracted to people of the same sex as they were assigned at birth (that is, transition would 'make them heterosexual') (Green, 1974, p xv). Yet the medicalised conflation of gender and sexuality was deeply fraught, and mid-20th-century clinicians saw it as equally essential to distinguish between prospective patients who were 'really' trans and those who were in fact 'merely' homosexual (Gill-Peterson, 2018, pp 80, 142). Similarly, while some 20th-century communities – particularly working-class, Black and Latine communities in the United States – understood little meaningful difference between 'gay' and 'trans' (Heyam, 2022, pp 116–19, 146–8), others from both camps sought to sharply demarcate the two experiences in the name of assimilation (Burns, 2018a, pp 30–1; Heyam, 2022, pp 146–8). Practitioners working with older trans people, then, should be prepared to encounter a range of diverse understandings of sexuality and gender – as intrinsically linked, or as sharply distinct – as well as a range of diverse attitudes towards LGB trans people and towards umbrella, solidarity-based groupings like 'LGBTQ+'.

Experiences of medical and social transition

These changing 20th-century conceptualisations of trans experience did not simply shape trans self-understanding in an abstract sense; they also had a very material impact on trans medical care. While transition-related medical care still has a great many shortcomings (Wright et al, 2021), those who transitioned during the 20th century (particularly before the 1990s) are likely to have experienced a specific set of harms. Adrienne Nash's account of her attempts to transition in the UK in the 1960s and 1970s includes disbelief, threats of arrest, offers of electroconvulsive and aversion therapy, religiously motivated refusals of treatment and forced resignation from her job (Nash, 2018); her experiences are echoed in many other, more large-scale surveys (Porter et al, 2016; Gill-Peterson, 2018; Pearce, 2018; Velocci, 2021). Indeed, Beans Velocci has shown that the 20th-century development of the gender identity clinic system was predicated on clinicians' distrust, disbelief and even fear of their trans patients: 'one could not be transsexual and also an expert on one's own needs' (Velocci, 2021, p 476). The legacy of such attitudes, whether for those who transitioned during this period or for those who simply lived through it, may include increased distrust of medical professionals; decision making oriented towards preserving privacy, even if this compromises care; and/or feelings of ambivalence about other trans people's more fluid or playful approaches to transition.

The historical production of realness: whose trans identities do we take seriously?

Thus far, I have argued that knowledge of trans history is valuable for practitioners working with older people insofar as it can facilitate understanding of diverse self-conceptualisations among older trans populations. Yet trans history has ethical and political value beyond its ability to mediate between different understandings and experiences of gender. At a deeper level, knowing more about trans history can also help us to think more critically about contemporary standards of what constitutes a 'real' or 'valid' trans identity – and thus to respond more openly to diverse trans experiences, developing a deeper respect for trans self-determination.

Contemporary anti-trans discourse is frequently oriented towards dismissing the ontological 'realness' of trans people: arguing that trans people are fake or disguised, or that the supposed 'truth' of our biological characteristics should always be given more weight than our identities (Williams, 2020; Heyam, 2022, pp 21–6). Consequently, trans politics often finds itself trapped into responding on those same ontological terms and engaging in strategies designed to prove the legitimacy of our identities (Catherwood, 2015, pp 43–4; Heyam, 2022). This frequently involves emphasising their *stability* (known from a young age, has not shifted, is not inherently fluid); their *medicalisation* (reliant on, and actively seeking, medical transition to relieve distress); their *separation of gender from other factors* (a desire for transition independent of, for example, sexuality or social roles); and their *stereotyped* nature (conforming closely to gender norms, often including heterosexuality, and necessarily troubled by non-binary identities) (Heyam,

2022, especially p 14). Evidencing these narrow yet pervasive criteria requires detailed, confessional personal testimony (Heyam, 2022, p 21).

The consequence of this ontologically oriented political struggle is that some trans experiences are typically treated as less valid, and therefore less worthy of respect, than others. Anyone whose identity is fluid, or their self-articulation recent; anyone who does not or cannot seek medical transition; anyone who experiences their gender as bound up with their sexuality, their role in society or other aspects of their life; anyone gender-non-conforming, especially non-heterosexual and/or non-binary people – all risk disbelief and disrespect of their identities and their requests for appropriate treatment such as correct pronouns.

Older trans people are arguably more likely to fall into many of these categories: they may have been prevented from articulating their trans experience early in life by stigma or lack of knowledge; may have previously de- or re-transitioned due to negative experiences of the kinds discussed earlier (Pearce, 2018); may be more likely to experience medical complications when seeking hormones or surgery, or to decide the risks of medical transition are not worth undertaking later in life (Pearce, 2018); may understand trans identities as related to sexuality or intersex traits, as discussed earlier; may find their access to gender-conforming presentation limited by an ageing body (Pearce, 2018); may, even if they do fulfil these narrow criteria of 'realness', be less willing to 'prove' them through personal testimony about their experiences owing to their experiences of the stealth imperative (Porter et al, p. 374); and may find that the propensity of all trans people to be 'not taken seriously within health and social care' can be 'multiplie[d]' by 'ageing and the prospect of conditions such as dementia' (Bailey, 2012, p 60). Consequently, an ethical commitment to trans allyship can be enhanced by appreciation of how these standards of 'realness' were historically produced. The two most significant factors which shaped them are both mid-20th-century phenomena: the emergence of the gender identity clinic (GIC) and its diagnostic criteria, and the concurrent development of the genre of trans memoir in print media.

The influential GICs of the mid-20th-century United States required patients to undergo extensive psychological assessment, and to provide extensive personal testimony, before being approved for treatment (Siatos et al, 2019, p 133). These assessments were aimed in part at detecting which patients were 'real' transsexuals and which were not and were predicated on an understanding of trans people as inherently untrustworthy (Catherwood, 2015, pp 44–5; Velocci, 2021). Diagnostic criteria included a 'strong, secure and consistent' gender identity (Gill-Peterson, 2018, p 147) and 'adherence to normative gender roles' (Velocci, 2021, p 463; see also Nash, 2018, p 48). As late as 1990, an article in the *British Journal of Psychiatry* described how clinicians' informal diagnostic criteria went beyond those in DSM-III to also include long-term stability ('age of onset'), separation of gender from other factors ('presence or absence of sexual arousal with cross dressing') and desire for full gender conformity ('a dislike of secondary sex characteristics') (Burns et al, 1990, p 265). The authors, among them a gender identity clinician, consider only trans people who fulfil these additional factors to be ' "core", "true" or "primary" transsexuals' (Burns et al, 1990, p 265).

These diagnostic criteria were helped on their way to becoming cultural consensus about what made a 'real' trans person by trans life narratives. Since the early 20th century, trans people in Europe and the United States have used self-disclosure – both book-length memoirs and first-person news interviews – to frame their identities in the public eye. These first-person narratives came to follow a familiar pattern, emphasising all the features previously outlined as characteristics of 'realness': a realisation in childhood led to a stable sense of trans identity characterised by a sense of 'wrongness' with one's body and a desire for medical transition which, once achieved, allowed the trans writer to live a stereotypical, gender-conforming life (Prosser, 1998; Catherwood, 2015, p 46; Jacques, 2017, pp 358–9). These memoirs often had a reciprocal relationship with medical diagnosis, both informed by and informing the narratives trans people gave to clinicians (Catherwood, 2015, p 47; Jacques, 2017, p 358). The centrality of personal testimony to both of these processes has led the cisgender public to expect, even feel entitled to, trans people's personal narratives (Catherwood, 2015, pp 51–2; Jacques, 2017, pp 360–7) – an effect only heightened by political contexts in which trans people's ontological 'realness' is under attack.

Conclusion

As this chapter has shown, the terminology and concepts of trans identity are dynamic, as is the nature of trans experience. The way older trans people understand and articulate their experiences of gender is likely to be diverse and in many cases to depart from normative present-day understanding. Knowledge of this conceptual and linguistic dynamism can facilitate fuller appreciation of the kinds of memories, habits and self-understandings that older trans people bring to their present-day experiences of care. Practitioners working with older trans people should therefore seek to develop their knowledge in this area and to apply it by recognising as paramount the self-definition of those they support, even if this conflicts with their own understanding of transness or that of others around them.

At the same time, knowledge of trans history can also help us to understand that contemporary criteria for what is considered a 'real' trans identity are neither objective nor politically neutral. On the contrary, they have been shaped by systems which were constructed in ways that encouraged disbelief of trans people and discouraged self-determination. Consequently, when anyone of any age expresses an aspect of their trans experience, practitioners should be critical of their instinctive response: to believe or disbelieve them, to respect their requests for how to be treated or to seek 'proof' in the form of personal testimony.

Though these recommendations are made with older trans people in mind, ultimately they apply to anyone invested in treating trans people with respect and care. Knowing that our understanding of what constitutes a 'real' trans identity is historically contingent, and that the way trans people understand and talk about their identities has shifted markedly during the 20th century, can help all practitioners to take more seriously and respond more openly to diverse gendered experiences and forms of self-identification. Vanessa D. Fabbre's call for gerontological practitioners to 'create meaningful collaborations with scholars and leaders in queer studies and gender-progressive movements' (2014, p 10) was timely in 2014 and is still more timely now. Historical scholarship must not remain isolated, framed as a recreational interest or an optional extra; it must be recognised, instead, as a valuable form of cultural competence and an essential contributor to ethical practice.

References

Amin, K. (2018) 'Glands, eugenics, and rejuvenation in *Man into Woman*: a biopolitical genealogy of transsexuality', *TSQ: Transgender Studies Quarterly*, 5(4): 589–605.

Bailey, L. (2012) 'Trans ageing: thoughts on a life course approach in order to better understand trans lives', in R. Ward, M. Sutherland and I. Rivers (eds) *Lesbian, Gay, Bisexual and Transgender Ageing: Biographical Approaches for Inclusive Care and Support*, London: Jessica Kingsley Publishers, pp 51–66.

Burns, A., Farrell, M. and Brown, J.C. (1990) 'Clinical features of patients attending a gender-identity clinic', *British Journal of Psychiatry*, 157: 265–8.

Burns, C. (2018a) 'Is there anyone else like me?', in C. Burns (ed) *Trans Britain: Our Journey from the Shadows*, London: Unbound, pp 23–38.

Burns, C. (ed) (2018b) *Trans Britain: Our Journey from the Shadows*, London: Unbound.

Catherwood, R. (2015) 'Coming *in*? The evolution of the transsexual memoir in the twenty-first century', *Genre*, 48(1): 35–71.

Ekins, R. and King, D. (2001) 'Pioneers of transgendering: the popular sexology of David O. Cauldwell', *International Journal of Transgenderism*, 5(2).

Fabbre, V.D. (2014) 'Gender transitions in later life: the significance of time in queer aging', *Journal of Gerontological Social Work*, 57(0): 161–75.

Fabbre, V.D. (2015) 'Gender transitions in later life: a queer perspective on successful aging', *The Gerontologist*, 55(1): 144–53.

Feinberg, L. (1994) *Transgender Warriors: Making History from Joan of Arc to Dennis Rodman*, Boston: Beacon Press.

Gill-Peterson, J. (2018) *Histories of the Transgender Child*, Minneapolis: University of Minnesota Press.

Green, R. (1974) *Sexual Identity Conflict in Children and Adults*, New York: Basic Books.

Griffiths, D.A. (2018) 'Diagnosing sex: intersex surgery and "sex change" in Britain 1930–1955', *Sexualities*, 21(3): 476–95.

Heyam, K. (2022) *Before We Were Trans: A New History of Gender*, London: Basic Books.

Jacques, J. (2017) 'Forms of resistance: uses of memoir, theory, and fiction in trans life writing', *Life Writing*, 14(3): 357–70.

Nash, A. (2018) 'The doctor won't see you now', in C. Burns (ed) *Trans Britain: Our Journey from the Shadows*, London: Unbound Burns, pp 39–50.

Pearce, R. (2018) 'Trans temporalities and non-linear ageing', in A. King, K. Almack, Y.-T. Suen and S. Westwood (eds) *Older Lesbian, Gay, Bisexual and Trans People: Minding the Knowledge Gaps*, London: Routledge, pp 61–74.

Porter, K.E., Brennan-Ing, M., Chang, S.C., dickey, l.m., Singh, A.A., Bower, K.L. et al (2016) 'Providing competent and affirming services for transgender and gender nonconforming older adults', *Clinical Gerontologist*, 39(5): 366–88.

Prosser, J. (1998) *Second Skins: Body Narratives of Transsexuality*, New York: Columbia University Press.

Raskolnikov, M., LaFleur, G. and Klosowska, A. (eds) (2021) *Trans Historical: Gender Plurality before the Modern*, Ithaca: Cornell University Press.

Siotos, C., Neira, P.M., Lau, B.D., Stone, J.P., Page, J., Rosson, G.D. et al (2019) 'Origins of gender affirmation surgery: the history of the first gender identity clinic in the United States at Johns Hopkins', *Annals of Plastic Surgery*, 83(2): 132–6.

Stryker, S. (2017) *Transgender History: The Roots of Today's Revolution* (2nd edn), New York: Seal Press.

Velocci, B. (2021) 'Standards of care: uncertainty and risk in Harry Benjamin's transsexual classifications', *TSQ: Transgender Studies Quarterly*, 8(4): 462–80.

Vicente, M.V. (2021) 'Transgender: a useful category? Or, how the historical study of "transsexual" and "transvestite" can help us rethink "transgender" as a category', *TSQ: Transgender Studies Quarterly*, 8(4): 426–42.

Williams, C. (2020) 'The ontological woman: a history of deauthentication, dehumanization, and violence', *The Sociological Review Monographs*, 68(4): 718–34.

Wright, T., Nicholls, E.J., Rodger, A.J., Burns, F.M., Weatherburn, P., Pebody, R. et al (2021) 'Accessing and utilising gender-affirming healthcare in England and Wales: trans and non-binary people's accounts of navigating gender identity clinics', *BMC Health Services Research*, 21(609): 1–11.

11

Reframing gender neutrality in dementia care cultures

Phil Harper

Introduction

Gender neutrality has been explored previously and presented as a negative way of erasing gender (Bartlett et al, 2018). In many cases, this is true. However, within dementia care, gender neutrality can also be a way of being inclusive of gender non-conforming individuals in care settings.

There are many different definitions of gender non-conformity due to the non-conformist nature of the term. In this chapter, I use the term 'gender non-conformity' to explain gender identities and expressions that do not conform to the dominant binary norms, such as 'man' or 'woman'. Gender non-conformity is not limited to non-binary genders; and while it is difficult to collect data on this population, it can be assumed that gender diverse individuals would make up the largest percentage of those who fall under the gender non-conforming category. The trans umbrella includes all individuals who do not identify with their sex assigned at birth. Gender non-conforming individuals often do identify under this umbrella, but this is not always the case, as some cisgender individuals (those who do identify as their sex assigned at birth) may also present their gender in a gender non-conforming way. While supporting gender non-conformity is an important consideration for the trans community, it is not only a trans issue.

While the chapter adopts the title 'Reframing gender neutrality in dementia care cultures', it does not intend to propose that those who are gender diverse or benefit from gender neutrality necessarily identify as gender neutral. However, a gender-neutral approach may be beneficial to those who do not conform to gender norms. Concerns about only adopting gender neutrality also have validity, and occur in many discussions within disability studies, given that disabled toilets are often gender neutral. Some individuals with disabilities commonly report that they are forced to push aside their gendered identity to have their needs met (Ghai, 2003). Therefore, care settings need to have plurality of gendered and gender-neutral support for those who would benefit from it.

It is difficult to estimate how many gender diverse and transgender individuals are living with dementia. As discussed in Chapter 1 of this book, statistics on gender identity have not historically been included in the UK census and in other population measures. The currently known demographic information on gender identity may be inaccurate due to confusing and misleading questions and the voluntary nature of these question (Guyan, 2022). This limits awareness around gender identity which may lead to erasure within care cultures and research. There is a need for more discussion around different approaches to supporting all those living with dementia who use care including gender non-conforming and gender diverse individuals.

Existing literature and best practice guidance, such as in Caceres (2019) and Harper (2019), states that care professionals need to be more aware of the needs of trans and gender diverse individuals living with dementia. However, this alone will not bring the change needed. In addition to education and awareness raising for care professionals, there needs to be some reflection on context such as organisational culture in settings where dementia care is provided and how this can be adapted to be more inclusive and empowering for those who are gender non-conforming.

Translocational positionality is a concept initially used within migration studies to explore the limitations of heuristic notions of identity, stating that our identity and positionality are situated within time and place (Anthias, 2008). This concept can inform methods used to explore intersectional experiences of identity, especially related to the fluidity of identity and self-efficacy in care settings, with a specific focus on how an individual's positionality may change if the setting is not inclusive. Organisational culture within a care setting commonly tends to erase gender-neutral expression and gender diverse identities due to a lack of awareness at all levels of the organisation (Sandberg, 2018).

This chapter will initially explore how the concept of translocational positionality can be adopted to understand experiences of trans and non-binary individuals living with dementia. I then continue to explore power, particularly adopting Michel Foucault's work on power and knowledge and other concepts of power dynamics within care settings. The chapter next examines the role of micro-aggression in care settings, particularly for trans and non-binary individuals living with dementia. Lastly, I propose recommendations for practice, especially stating the need for a pluralistic approach to dementia care, which is inclusive for cisgender and trans and non-binary individuals in care settings.

Translocational positionality, intersectionality and identity

Rogers and Ahmed (2017) apply the concept of translocational positionality to sexual orientation and gender identity, particularly emphasising the rejection of the binary for gender diverse individuals and how this is evidence of the fluid nature of identity based on historical documentation and social context. This adoption of translocational positionality helps to provide a framework to understand how an individual's relationship with their identity, especially gender identity, might change based on the setting and cultures adopted by that setting over time.

It is important to note that gender diversity is not new; however, current labels and names of specific identities might be more recent (Rogers and Ahmed, 2017). Therefore, identifying and supporting individuals, particularly older gender non-conforming individuals, can be challenging. According to the notions of translocational positionality, this could impact an individual's association with their identity and impact professionals' lack of knowledge around specific needs in care settings, especially for those who have limited understanding of different gender identities. This is one of the reasons why gender non-conformity is a useful identifier when exploring the care needs of older individuals, as it has been historically recognised more than other identities such as non-binary. However, this does not mean that it is understood by staff in care settings due to ongoing limited understanding of gender expression and diversity.

Translocational positionality provides a useful intersectional framework that allows us to understand the complexity of oppression and discrimination. Crenshaw (1989) originally introduced the concept of intersectionality based on Black women's experiences of discrimination, focusing particularly on the overlap between gender and race, which compound to create unique challenges and forms of discrimination. Translocational positionality allows us to understand how an individual's identity is viewed in time and space and therefore how intersections of identity are fluid and may change, leading to changing needs over time. For example, in queer spaces and at a time when understanding of gender identity is developing, an individual may feel more comfortable presenting in a gender non-conforming way. This may intersect with an individual's age, ethnicity or religion. Where the environment is affirming, an individual may not feel the need to regularly highlight their gender identity and any relevant needs as it would be perceived that they are already known. However, in less affirming environments, an individual may need to disclose their identity more often to avoid potential challenges, such as being misgendered by other residents or staff. An individual may also choose not to disclose their gender identity and choose to hide their gender non-conformity, leading to a perceived lower intersectional or compounding layer of identity. These examples demonstrate how translocational positionality can provide a useful framework for understanding intersectionality and how the fluid nature of identity and positionality can impact how we consider and recognise intersections in identity.

Dementia care settings and power

Foucault, a French sociologist, often explored power in relation to identity. In Foucault's archaeology of knowledge (Foucault, 1970), this can be easily applied to the separate theory of translocational positionality. Foucault states that historical discourse can influence current knowledge and that knowledge is fluid in its nature based on developments in knowledge and understanding. This concept of subjective truth and discursive power is relevant to care cultures when exploring inclusive language and gender identity. As previously stated, the existence of diverse gender identities is not new; however, the label or name used to describe identities may be more recent. Therefore, we need to consider the language used and how a person may identify with a more historical but less accurate identity. For example, an older individual who was assigned male at birth and is gender non-conforming may identify as gay, as this was the most common and known LGBTQ+ identity when they came out. Therefore, we need to consider all identities when working towards inclusivity, taking a pluralistic approach to gender identity and expression, enabling gender neutrality and enabling binary gender expression.

Foucault explored surveillance and self-regulation and how these forms of disciplinary power operate in modern society. He used the analogy of the panopticon, a circular prison with a central watcher in the middle, designed by Jeremy Bentham. This is an effective prison design as prisoners can be watched at any one time from the centre, and it has been observed that prisoners start to self-regulate their behaviour due to fear of being caught breaking rules. Foucault applied this idea of self-regulation to wider society, where the watchers at the centre are those responsible for promoting the dominant discourse (Foucault, 2012). Individuals therefore start to behave and conform to societal norms based on the available discourse of the time, which, as previously stated, is historical and subjective in nature. This is evident in the theory of heteronormativity, in which LGBTQ+ individuals often try and conform to heterosexual norms and ideals due to society championing heterosexuality (Butler, 1999). Based on these analyses, we can start to see how care cultures can have a significant impact on an individual who is LGBTQ+, specifically trans and gender non-conforming individuals and their sense of identity.

Heteronormative imagery and language in care settings is driven by dominant discourse, such as same sex, cisgender couples displayed on posters, and care staff making heteronormative assumptions when asking if an individual has a partner. This discourse reinforces the heteronormative demographic, resulting in LGBTQ+, specifically gender non-conforming individuals not feeling accepted and/or adapting their behaviours to fit this discourse, potentially including hiding their identity. This example demonstrates the power that a care culture can have over an individual and the importance of conveying inclusive messages within care cultures.

Some individuals receiving care and support may experience internalised prejudice. Internalised prejudice is where individuals adopt negative and oppressive views and opinions of their own identity (Cornish, 2012). An example of this could be when a trans individual contributes to dominant transphobic discourse around toilet use and where constant exposure to this rhetoric leads to internalisation by individuals impacted by rhetoric. Applying these concepts to translocational positionality illustrates how an individual's self-regulation and internalised prejudice can cause them to become disassociated with their identity, hide their authentic selves and even contribute to oppressive power dynamics.

In care settings, there are clear power dynamics, especially between the individual being cared for and the professional or worker providing care. According to Lawler (2008), in Western society, particularly, we have a choice to be governed by societal power dynamics. However, in care settings, an individual may have less autonomy over their life and everyday decisions (Harper, 2020). Power dynamics may become emphasised, especially for those who have limited mental capacity.

Lawler (2008) observes how more covert and subtle forms of power are more effective and can be hard to address when attempting to have autonomy over our lives. Individuals living with dementia are often reliant on care professionals to provide gender-affirming care in addition to meeting their physical needs, for example through actions such as the application of personal make-up. This is especially prevalent for those who break societal norms regarding gender expression, for example those who are assigned male at birth but wear make-up to express a trans or non-conforming identity. Professionals and care workers in care settings need to consider how they will challenge and transverse these power dynamics, especially for LGBTQ+ individuals who face challenges that are different from their cisgendered and heterosexual peers, alongside the intersectional challenges from being gender non-conforming and living with dementia (Borrill, 2000). Dementia may impact on loss of voice based on ableist assumptions about an individual's capacity (Borrill, 2000). This is a form of double jeopardy for gender diverse individuals who feel erased and subsequently retreat back into the metaphorical closet or, where this is not possible, may impact on their self-efficacy. The role of advocacy from those who understand the needs of the individual is vital in ensuring that their voice is heard, especially when a person has limited or fluctuating mental capacity.

Dementia further intersects with diverse gender identities in other unique ways. It is common for gender neutrality or non-conformity to be pathologised within the care of a person living with dementia (Sandberg, 2018). This often happens as a heteronormative lens is adopted in which non-conforming ways of presenting gender are attributed as a symptom of dementia rather than being seen as intrinsic to an individual's sense of self (Sandberg, 2018). This pathologisation can often create complexities around breaking down power dynamics in dementia care. For example, if an individual living with dementia presents in a gender-neutral or non-conforming way, care staff may take it on themselves to 'support' the individual in dressing based on the care professional's assumptions about their gender, which is not necessarily the gender the individual identifies with or wants to express as.

Recent research has suggested that dementia might help an individual be their authentic self by freeing them from some of the power structures discussed (Silverman and Baril, 2023). For example, dementia may mean that an individual experiences more congruence with their self-identified gender than with their sex assigned at birth. One example from Silverman and Baril's (2023) research was a trans man living with dementia who does not have a penis but who believed they had a penis when using the toilet. This therefore demonstrates that gender is more than just the physical body, and dementia may lead to an individual associating closer to their self-identified gender and in a more fluid way based on how an individual relates to their gender identity. This demonstrates the need for power dynamics within care settings to be critically analysed and for care professionals and workers to always start with how an individual seeks to express themselves and their identity. I therefore suggest that care professionals should think beyond sex and consider other gender identities and the physical needs an individual may have, for example not assume toilet habits for a non-binary person living with dementia based on their sex assigned at birth.

Dementia can lead to other complexities when providing affirming care. It is common for a person living with dementia to fall back to previous points in time (Andrews, 2015). This can cause some fear for individuals living with dementia, especially gender non-conforming individuals who drop back to a less accepting era. This scenario can also create challenges where care staff, due to unequal power dynamics, might be perceived as those *in* power. For example, a gender non-conforming individual might drop back to a point where being gender non-conforming was not socially accepted. Care staff wearing uniforms could invoke fear of the police or similar authorities and fear of disclosing their gender identity and/or expression. These are complex issues for care staff to navigate in their consideration of the individual and organisational power that they hold. Considering Foucault's adoption of the panopticon as previously discussed can often help understand power dynamics and internalised pressures caused by authoritarian figures (Foucault, 2012). Those living with dementia may have memory concerns, and such affirming discourse might need to be constant/repeated to remind the individuals of the accepting care culture.

The emotional labour of being in a heteronormative setting is another consideration. Health and social care environments can be a scary and difficult setting even without the added complexities of heteronormativity and a cognitive condition such as dementia. According to Vincent (2020), non-binary and gender non-conforming individuals often fear healthcare and heteronormative settings, and in accordance with the concept of translocational positionality, non-binary and gender non-conforming individuals' behaviours change within such settings. For example, non-binary people in less accepting environments often become less visible and use identity descriptors that are more widely understood. Therefore, in a less inclusive care setting, a gender non-conforming individual living with dementia may decide to present in a more conforming manner, to avoid negative reactions and treatment, which in turn may lead to the erasure of an individual's identity and personhood.

Micro-aggressions and the role of language in dementia care settings

Part of understanding the needs of trans people living with dementia is being self-aware about how subtleties in our language and behaviour may lead to a less than supportive environment for an individual. This intersectional awareness helps to contribute to a supportive environment and inclusive care culture for trans individuals, especially gender non-conforming individuals living with dementia. As explored previously, translocational positionality can be defined as positionality in the context of time and place and, therefore, impacts how an individual views their identity (Rogers and Ahmed, 2017). By reviewing language and subtleties in our practice, we can hopefully create an inclusive environment that enables gender non-conforming individuals to be their authentic selves.

The concept of micro-aggressions was initially explored in relation to racism (Pierce et al, 1977). The concept was developed to include other minority groups, including LGBTQ+ communities. Vaccaro and Koob (2019) also state that it is only very recently that scholars have started to explore intersectionality when exploring micro-aggressions, for example where individuals have two or more characteristics that can be discriminated against. LGBTQ+ micro-aggressions in dementia care have been briefly explored previously; however, due to the lack of focus on intersectionality when exploring care cultures (Vaccaro and Koob, 2019), this is often only briefly mentioned as part of wider research or in opinion articles, such as in Harper (2019). Gaining an in-depth understanding of how micro-aggressions operate helps create inclusive care cultures that can meet the needs of gender diverse and trans individuals, especially those individuals living with dementia.

Nadal et al (2010) provide examples of LGBTQ+ micro-aggressions including terminology that discriminates against a LGBTQ+ person, the enforcement of heterosexual norms, disregarding LGBTQ+ people's individual experiences and not accepting that an LGBTQ+ person has specific care needs. These micro-aggressions, however, interact with dementia symptoms in a unique way. The enforcement of heterosexual norms has already been discussed previously through the concept of heteronormativity and is a theme that threads itself throughout the other examples discussed subsequently.

The impact of incorrect terminology and language

The positive use of language is essential in enabling a trans person to feel validated (Ansara and Hegarty, 2014). The overfocus on the gender binary is common, particularly in healthcare settings (Harper, 2020); however, this is also evident in other care settings and cultures. This can provide an unwelcoming environment, particularly for gender diverse individuals who may not identify with the gender binary. Some examples of micro-aggressions include the use of incorrect terminology or providing gender binary options limited to bathrooms, admission forms and specific activities including social events.

According to Kitwood (1997), professionals often unintentionally cause harm by overlooking a person's social needs; this concept is known as malignant social psychology (MSP). Labelling a person is potentially an example of this MSP. According to Richards and Barker (2013), sexuality and gender identity are complicated, and labelling does not allow for the individuality of sexuality and gender identity. Not every non-binary or gender non-conforming individual presents in the same way, which demonstrates the need to break away from these labels and boxes and treat everybody as an individual. This is essential for a person living with dementia, as everyone's journey and symptoms are different. Kitwood (1997) uses the following quote to emphasise this: 'When you've met one person with dementia, you've met one person with dementia.' By treating every individual in a person-centred way, we can ensure that individual presentation and expression are encouraged, especially when an individual expresses themselves in a gender non-conforming way. When providing care for a trans and gender non-conforming person living with dementia, we must not enforce our gender norms on the individual and assume the individual's needs and behaviours, as a person may have different needs and wants than what you understand. Older individuals might be more comfortable with terms that were more prevalent when they came out; and whoever they are, they might present aspects of gender in a different way than the norm. This demonstrates the need for a person-centred approach that does not erase individual needs and differences.

Professional working with an LGBTQ+ person living with dementia

According to Witten (2015), older LGBTQ+ individuals fear health and care services, often due to professionals' lack of understanding about their specific needs. This fear is especially prevalent within the trans community (Witten, 2015). Some examples of the lack of understanding have already been discussed, for example in language when professionals misgender a person who is trans or gender non-conforming. The fear of developing or showing symptoms of dementia often accompanies the stigma attached to the disease. Trans people, especially gender non-conforming individuals, may avoid seeking formal diagnosis when experiencing memory concerns. As stated previously, the inclusion of trans- and non-binary-affirming imagery and literature, especially in care settings, can help a person feel validated and may also communicate to individuals that that setting understands their specific needs. Examples of affirming imagery and literature could include images of gender non-conforming individuals on posters and trans health advice leaflets. Providing dementia literature and support in LGBTQ+ settings and centres may increase awareness and provide support in a safe environment for individuals to be prepared for getting older. This is particularly relevant for trans and gender non-conforming individuals, where protecting their gender identity and non-heteronormative expression is important when entering heteronormative care cultures.

Harper (2019) notes that non-heteronormative partners of a person living with dementia in health and social care settings are also commonly overlooked and not recognised as important. This can include partners who are gender non-conforming themselves. Harper (2019) argues that partners and family members hold essential expertise about the wants and wishes of the individual in care settings. It is common, especially for a single trans or gender non-conforming individual, to have close friends and significant others which constitute a 'family of choice' (Donovan et al, 2001). A chosen family, opposed to a biological family, is one that an individual has chosen to be around them. As illustrated in other chapters, there are known conflicts between these families of choice and biological family members. It is common for trans individuals to have a closer chosen family due to high levels of rejection and lack of awareness of gender needs from their biological family. These situations are described by Hafford-Letchfield et al in Chapter 9 in this book regarding social support. This may be especially likely where trans and gender diverse individuals have come out in later years and decisions around gender-affirming care need to be made (Barret et al, 2015). This demonstrates the need for a diverse view of family and recognition of close friends in care planning and delivery for enabling care settings to be inclusive of all genders and gender expressions. Empowering family of choice and non-heteronormative partners, especially those who also express in a gender non-confirming way, is an especially effective way of breaking down unequal power dynamics between care staff and professionals and individuals receiving care. It also ensures cultures are inclusive of those who are LGBTQ+, especially transgender and gender non-conforming individuals. The role of an advocate might also be essential in ensuring that the needs of an individual are met when there is conflict or a lack of 'chosen family', especially when mental capacity fluctuates.

Professionals may pathologise gender expression by dismissing the specific needs of a gender non-conforming individual living with dementia. Gender expression is an important way for an LGBTQ+ individual, especially one who is gender diverse, to express their gender and selves. Clothing and make-up, for example, are ways an individual can express themselves in a gender non-conforming way which may require support from care professionals. This could be an example of a specific power dynamic a care professional can hold over trans, especially gender non-conforming, individuals. A lack of awareness around how a person might want to dress and therefore not supporting someone to dress in a way that is in line with their wants and wishes could also be deemed a micro-aggression and shows a lack of respect for the individual's specific needs. An added complexity is that an individual with dementia may not be able to communicate their wishes clearly due to their dementia or due to fear, as discussed previously. This is where accepting family, friends and partners are essential advocates, supporting the individual to be their authentic self and ensuring that the care setting meets the needs of their loved one.

Recommendations for practice

In care settings, gender non-conformity needs to be recognised as a valid gender expression which can become complicated or compromised due to cognitive decline. While knowing an individual's medical needs is essential, understanding an individual's personal identity and wishes is also essential when providing person-centred care. Therefore, care professionals need to know an individual's gender identity and expression and support this vital aspect of who they are.

In relation to gender non-conforming individuals, this would mean ensuring that care settings and cultures are affirming. Considering Foucault's panopticon and power dynamics, care professionals need to ensure that those in care do not feel pressured into going back into the closet. This can be supported by having regular gender-affirming conversations, including local and national pride events reflecting wider societal change. Inclusive posters co-created with and specially for the trans and non-binary community showing same-sex partners, gender non-conformity and diverse individuals also help to create a welcoming environment for all members of the LGBTQ+ community. While the goal is to make the whole care setting inclusive, this is not always realistic due to factors outside the care setting's control, such as the views and behaviours of other residents. However, it remains essential, and it is an ethical duty of care for professionals to provide safe spaces that are affirming; this extends beyond an older person's bedroom or private space. The provision of safe spaces within heteronormative environments can help to minimise triggering any previous experience of hostility and minimise potential for divisive experiences currently reflected in society.

Care staff should feel empowered to challenge heteronormative and cisnormative assumptions and practices through the establishment of a change organisational culture. A diverse workforce is one element in which care settings can be inclusive through positive representation and upholding the value of everyone's lived experiences (Cohen et al, 2002). Representation within a diverse workforce can also support breaking down power dynamics within the setting. The LGBTQ+ community is not homogenous, and there is intersection and potential complexity of gender and sexual identities (Caceres, 2019). LGBTQ+ staff may themselves not be tuned into microaggressions, nor is it their sole responsibility. Finding ways of engaging and supporting gender diverse staff will however contribute to better care culture.

Care professionals need to become more aware of the needs of a trans person living with dementia, especially gender non-confirming individuals and the people closest to them. Care professionals should be encouraged to identify the conflicts between families and the wishes of a gender diverse or trans individual lacking capacity and, if possible, should involve the people closest to them, which may not always be biological family. Where this is not possible, an independent mental capacity advocate should be appointed. This will ensure decisions are in the individual's best interests, which may not align with the perspectives of those who do not understand or approve of an individual's sexuality or gender identity. Education around advance care planning and lasting power of attorney would also help support a gender diverse or trans individual's wishes to be met if they develop dementia. Specialist legal advice on LGBTQ+ human rights may help create awareness of the importance of this, especially for trans and gender diverse individuals where there may be more conflict around their self-identified gender.

Gender neutrality, when adopted in a pluralistic approach alongside gendered language, enables care settings and cultures to be inclusive of all gender identities and sexualities. For example, a way to avoid using incorrect pronouns is by adopting gender-neutral pronouns if a person's gender identity is not known. Examples of gender-neutral pronouns are 'they' and 'them'. Using these pronouns can lead to better inclusion, especially for a person with dementia, who can present with confusion and possibly fear of coming out in a heteronormative setting. Gender neutrality, however, should always be used in a pluralistic way, and gendered language should be used when pronouns and gender identity are known. Including these choices in assessment/care plans is to ask how somebody would like to be addressed; we often ask this in dementia care but forget that this can also help with gender identity, not just a preferred name. Alongside asking, we can also include in the conversation the acceptance of different genders and provide our own pronouns to hopefully break down unequal power dynamics and show that the culture in the setting is inclusive. In contrast to previous suggestions that gender neutrality is the erasure of gender, adopting gender neutrality can support the expression of gender non-conforming identities. Therefore, adopting a pluralistic approach where gendered language and gender neutrality can both be used by professionals is an important way of supporting all gender identities and expressions. I conclude this chapter by asking the reader to rethink gender neutrality and consider it as a tool to help with inclusion in dementia care settings.

Summary learning points

- A holistic approach to support, where individuals are celebrated rather than managed, is needed as a means of promoting ethical and inclusive practices and moving away from the over-pathologisation of dementia through a strength-based approach that recognises the diverse identities of those living with dementia.
- Professionals need to reflect on the power and authority that may impact how gender non-conforming individuals with dementia ask for support with their gender expression. Care settings where people are living with dementia should reflect on the impact of heteronormativity and cisnormativity, considering how they can be visibly inclusive and support those who may fear having their identity and needs ignored.
- Give attention to recognising and responding to reduce micro-aggressions in practice in relation to gender identity and expression.
- Consider advocacy for trans, non-binary and gender non-conforming individuals living with dementia, ensuring that their subjective needs are met, supported by good practice in documentation and care planning.
- Adopting a person-centred and holistic approach can be enriched through a pluralist approach, including both gendered support and gender-neutral approaches.

References

Andrews, J. (2015) *Dementia: The One-Stop Guide; Practical Advice for Families, Professionals, and People Living with Dementia and Alzheimer's Disease*, London: Profile Books.

Ansara, Y.G. and Hegarty, P. (2014) 'Methodologies of misgendering: recommendations for reducing cisgenderism in psychological research', *Feminism & Psychology*, 24(2): 259–70.

Anthias, F. (2008) 'Thinking through the lens of translocational positionality: an intersectionality frame for understanding identity and belonging', *Translocations: Migration and Social Change*, 4(1): 5–20.

Barrett, C., Crameri, P., Lambourne, S., Latham, J.R. and Whyte, C. (2015) 'Understanding the experiences and needs of lesbian, gay, bisexual and trans Australians living with dementia, and their partners', *Australasian Journal on Ageing*, 34: 34–8.

Bartlett, R., Gjernes, T., Lotherington, A.T. and Obstefelder, A. (2018) 'Gender, citizenship and dementia care: a scoping review of studies to inform policy and future research', *Health & Social Care in the Community*, 26(1): 14–26.

Borrill, J. (2000) 'Listening to dementia', *Mental Health Nursing*, 20(4): 23.

Butler, J. (1999) *Gender Trouble: Feminism and the Subversion of Identity*, New York: Routledge.

Caceres, B.A. (2019) 'Care of LGBTQ older adults: what geriatric nurses must know', *Geriatric Nursing*, 40(3): 342–3.

Cohen, J.J., Gabriel, B.A. and Terrell, C. (2002) 'The case for diversity in the health care workforce', *Health Affairs*, 21(5): 90–102.

Cornish, M.J. (2012) 'The impact of internalised homophobia and coping strategies on psychological distress following the experience of sexual prejudice', PhD thesis, University of Hertfordshire.

Crenshaw, K. (1989) 'Demarginalizing the intersection of race and sex: a Black feminist critique of antidiscrimination doctrine, feminist theory and antiracist politics', *University of Chicago Legal Forum*, 1989(1): 139–67.

Donovan, C., Heaphy, B. and Weeks, J. (2003) *Same Sex Intimacies: Families of Choice and Other Life Experiments*. Routledge.

Foucault, M. (1970) 'The archaeology of knowledge', *Social Science Information*, 9(1): 175–85.

Foucault, M. (2012) *Discipline and Punish: The Birth of the Prison*, New York: Vintage.

Ghai, A. (2003) *(Dis)embodied Form: Issues of Disabled Women*, New Delhi: Har-Anand Publications.

Guyan, K. (2022) *Queer Data: Using Gender, Sex and Sexuality Data for Action*, London: Bloomsbury Academic.

Harper, P. (2019) 'How healthcare professionals can support older LGBTQ+ people living with dementia', *Nursing Older People* 117. DOI: 10.7748/nop.2019.e1115

Harper, P. (2020) 'Transgender and gender non-conforming peoples experience of being admitted to hospital', *International Journal of Research and Innovation in Social Science* 4(6): 351–6.

Kitwood, T. (1997) 'The experience of dementia', *Aging & Mental Health*, 1(1): 13–22.

Lawler, S. (2008) *Identity: Sociological Perspectives*, Cambridge: Polity.

Lawler, S. (2013) *Identity: Sociological Perspectives*, John Wiley & Sons.

Nadal, K.L., Rivera, D.P., Corpus, J.H. and Sue, D.W. (2010) 'Sexual orientation and transgender microaggressions', in D.W. Sue (ed) *Microaggressions and Marginality: Manifestation, Dynamics, and Impact*, Hoboken: Wiley, pp 217–40.

Pierce, C.M., Carew, J.V., Pierce-Gonzalez, D. and Wills, D. (1977) 'An experiment in racism: TV commercials', *Education and Urban Society*, 10(1): 61–87.

Richards, C. and Barker, M. (2013) *Sexuality and Gender for Mental Health Professionals: A Practical Guide*, London: Sage.

Rogers, M. and Ahmed, A. (2017) 'Interrogating trans and sexual identities through the conceptual lens of translocational positionality', *Sociological Research Online*, 22(1): 81–94.

Sandberg, L.J. (2018) 'Dementia and the gender trouble? Theorising dementia, gendered subjectivity and embodiment', *Journal of Aging Studies*, 45: 25–31.

Silverman, M. and Baril, A. (2023) '"We have to advocate so hard for ourselves and our people": caring for a trans or non-binary older adult with dementia', *LGBTQ+ Family: An Interdisciplinary Journal*, 19(3): 187–210.

Vaccaro, A. and Koob, R.M. (2019) 'A critical and intersectional model of LGBTQ microaggressions: toward a more comprehensive understanding', *Journal of Homosexuality*, 66(10): 1317–44.

Vincent, B. (2020) *Non-binary Genders: Navigating Communities, Identities, and Healthcare*, Bristol: Policy Press.

Witten, T.M. (2015) 'Elder transgender lesbians: exploring the intersection of age, lesbian sexual identity, and transgender identity', *Journal of Lesbian Studies*, 19(1): 73–89.

12

End-of-life care needs and considerations for older trans people

Kathryn Almack, Olivia Warnes and Eloise Kane

Introduction

In the UK and around the world, there are likely to be increasing numbers of trans people who will need care in late age and at the end of life, yet there is a paucity of research which addresses their specific needs and concerns. This is important, given some evidence which has found trans older adults are likely to have significantly poorer physical health, higher rates of disability and depressive symptomatology and greater perceived stress than the cisgender LGB older adult participants (Fredriksen-Goldsen et al, 2014; Reisner et al, 2016). Witten (2016) has written extensively on transgender ageing and reports on the invisibility and family isolation that trans older adults may face. Such factors can impact on life expectancy, and there are many nuanced considerations for trans older people at the end of life that we will address in this commentary, drawing on existing research and illustrated by quotes taken from our own studies. We report on research that has addressed the needs and concerns of trans people within the broader field of the end-of-life care for LGBT+ people as well as more recent work specifically focused on trans end-of-life care, and we conclude with some recommendations for future research.

Trans end-of-life care

Trans people are not routinely included in health service demographics, and as such it is very hard to be precise about the number of people from the trans and gender diverse community that will need end-of-life care. According to the 2021 UK census estimated that there were around 262,000 people openly willing to state that they had a gender identity different from their sex assigned at birth. The National Palliative and End of Life Care Partnership (2021) define end-of-life care as patients who are likely to die within the next 12 months (although in practice, end-of-life care is often delivered in the last weeks of life). The Partnership draws on the World Health Organization definition of palliative care as 'an approach that improves the quality of life of patients and their families who are facing problems associated with life-threatening illness' (2021, p 38). End-of-life and palliative care aims to be person-centred, which means identifying and meeting a person's individual physical, psychological, social and spiritual needs. This is often referred to as 'holistic care', which is a central tenet of end-of-life and palliative care. In England, for example, this ethos is reflected in the National Health Service's development of the Comprehensive Personalised Care Model, designed to enhance personalised palliative and end-of-life care to support increased choice and control at the end of life and provide a better experience of care. This includes earlier identification of people who are likely to die within the next 12 months; better conversations for people to identify their needs and preferences, and to share this information with those involved in their care; and integrated services which wrap around people. However, person-centred care can fail to consider the nuances of needs presented by trans people, in part due to a lack of research in this field.

In the last years of life, individuals and those important to them may need access to multiple services across different settings. It is important that trans people and those close to them feel safe in approaching services for assistance: if they are not confident about services or staff, they may not seek support. The care of the dying is said to be a good indicator of the care for all sick and vulnerable people. It is a crucial time to deliver good-quality care to enable individuals to die in comfort and with dignity because, to paraphrase Dame Cicely Saunders (recognised as the founder of the modern hospice movement), how someone dies remains a lasting memory for the individual's friends, family and the staff involved. All individuals should be afforded the same standard of care, compassion and dignity through life and at the end of life, but inequalities in terms of access to services, lack of confidence to access services and discriminatory attitudes still exist (see, for example, Stinchcombe et al, 2017; Gott et al, 2020; Rowley et al, 2021; Koffman et al, 2023). Addressing the distinctly complex and multiple needs of trans people holds the potential to develop non-discriminatory services that will benefit all.

Research relating to trans end-of-life care

A systematic review (Harding et al, 2012) of peer reviewed research published between 1990 and 2010 specifically addressing palliative and end-of-life care in LGBT+ populations identified only 12 relevant papers (the criteria excluded papers not published in English). No papers were found that reported specifically on transgender people's experiences. A more recent review of UK literature on LGBT health inequalities in later life identifies a lacuna in evidence about the lives of trans people

(Kneale et al, 2021). However, since the Harding et al (2012) systematic review, research exploring LGBT end-of-life care experiences and needs has grown significantly (Rosa et al, 2023). The bulk of the research (in English) comes from Australia, Canada, the United States and the UK (see, for example, Almack et al, 2010; Cartwright et al, 2012; Rawling, 2012; Lawton et al, 2013; and Bristowe et al, 2018). However, the identification of the particular needs of trans older adults at the end of life may be subsumed into research regarding LGBT+ older adults more generally (Almack and King, 2019). This research often involves only a few trans men and trans women, and even fewer non-binary people.

For many trans people, their life experiences have included facing situations/encounters where they are likely to feel particularly vulnerable with understandable fears about discriminatory attitudes. Willis et al identify this as 'trans precarity' (see Willis et al, 2021, for further discussion). While all older adults facing illness and frailty towards the end of life may experience or anticipate some vulnerability when becoming dependent on others to meet their care needs, these feelings are likely to be particularly acute for trans individuals with additional anxieties related to a lifetime legacy of experiences of exclusion, discrimination or isolation. In relation to end-of-life care, Witten (2014) describes a triple set of challenges for trans people on the basis of ageism, the stigma attached to trans identities and the impact of living with a chronic condition or terminal illness. Such anxieties detract from a dying person and their carers being able to have peace of mind towards the end of life and having a good experience of end-of-life care. To be living with a life-limiting condition and/or coming towards the end of life can be socially excluding experiences without the further layers of exclusion that trans people may face at these times. Also of relevance here are issues of finances and living circumstances when coming towards the end of life (see Rowley Richards et al, 2021), which can impact on choices at the end of life. There is some evidence to suggest financial and socioeconomic insecurity impact disproportionally on trans people across the life course (Carpenter et al, 2020). We are only just beginning to understand how the context of poverty and deprivation shapes experiences at the end of life, let alone think about intersections with other aspects of people's identity. Additional issues include the physical impacts of ageing as well as the side effects of end-of-life care treatments, which may, first, lead to changes to an individual's physical appearance, which may be particularly difficult for someone who is trans, and secondly interfere with the pharmacotherapy involved in transitioning. It is important to remember that non-binary people may also have pharmacological treatment. We currently have very little research on the long-term health outcomes in this group, and this should be an area of future focus.

Trans people frequently face difficult decisions about what to say and to whom about their gender identity. Encountering a wide range of staff means repeatedly having to assess whether it is safe to 'out' themselves. They might come across inconsistencies in their medical records and have to fight to rectify this and anticipate or wonder how to challenge inappropriate care. Facing such issues can be exhausting, especially if you are already feeling ill or vulnerable. An example of good practice is illustrated in a quote from the 'Last outing' study (Almack, 2019), from an interview with a trans woman facing a terminal diagnosis:

> 'I was in hospital and somebody came along and drew the curtains and I thought oh shit what's going on. She was the ward secretary or something, and she said "I'm having problems matching up your file, Ivy, because you say you've had [name of condition] but we've got no record. The nearest we've got is a person with your same date of birth but a different name." I was able to say "Yes, that used to be me." So she said "OK, that's fine I can combine them now." And I thought that's really enlightened, she hadn't even used my past name but treated me for who I am now. A little bit of thought works wonders.' (Ivy, 67, trans lesbian)

This is indicative of what good practice looks like in end-of-life care: Ivy had more peace of mind once she knew that her records had been matched up and also felt reassured that this had been well handled by the staff member. Further work has established the importance of keeping information such as this private in a care setting and ensuring that staff have the confidence and understanding to approach these situations sensitively (Hospice UK, 2023).

Service providers often have even less knowledge about the issues relating to trans people than those relating to LGB individuals. It is important to separate out sexual orientation from gender identity although equally important to note that there may be additional barriers for a trans person who is also LGB+. Trans people can face particular challenges if they have to negotiate intimate care with care staff who may not be aware of their particular needs:

> 'I've always been very private. As a male to female trans (person) still having beard growth, this would be an area of care I'd need and want to continue if I am became incapacitated … unable to shave and apply hair growth inhibitor myself. And other intimate care – dilation and routine douching to keep the vagina clear of possible infections. Hormone therapy is necessary until death and I'd want that to continue.' (Quote from the 'Last outing' study, Almack, 2019)

Trans people will be alert to nuanced responses upon disclosing information about their gender identity. As noted, every encounter with someone new can be accompanied by concerns about how that individual will respond to information disclosed. As a participant in Pang and colleagues' study (2019, p 49) reports, responses may not be blatantly discriminatory but there can still be "subtle Othering that goes on ... if your body's different you have no choice. If you have a nurse there or personal support worker, they're going to know at some point. So, there's a vulnerability around that."

Trans and gender diverse people should be empowered to have conversations about their body, needs and boundaries when they need to, so they can feel safe and comfortable with the care they receive. Any points of disclosure can be critical one-chance moments – if not met positively, this can be a missed opportunity to build up caring relationships and to get to know the whole person, which is central to holistic end-of-life care. Willis et al (2021, p 2808) note the importance of 'responding affirmingly to the successes' experienced by trans people 'in developing confidence to be and present as themselves across their lifetime while living in cisnormative social environments'.

It is additionally important to be aware of the diversity among trans people: some will have spent most of their lives with a gender identity and body other than the one assigned at birth, while for others this may be a relatively recent transition. Some may refer to 'transgender' as an aspect of their status or history, rather than part of their current identity. Others may identify as non-binary. Research has noted that for some trans older people, transitions, at a stage in life more commonly regarded as later life, are not uniformly experienced; indeed, later life may bring significant new beginnings. Initiatives to promote end-of-life care planning conversations among trans older adults must be sensitive to these (Pang et al, 2019; Willis et al, 2021). Pang and colleagues (2019) further note the roles of family, friends and community in the lives of trans participants, which can present both challenges and opportunities for fostering supportive connections for later life. Social support is important to consider in terms of networks to support trans people as health needs intensify, and evidence suggests that formal healthcare and support provision are likely play an important role in the later and end-of-life care for many (Catlett et al, 2023). For some trans people, experiences of marginalisation and discrimination over their life course may mean that they are socially isolated:

> Society, family values and lack of information when growing up meant I kept my real self hidden and has caused problems throughout my life. I feel I've lived a false life. Lonely, secretive, isolated, not

wanting to open myself up to others and find it difficult to make close friendships. (Trans participant; survey comment from the 'Last outing' study, Almack, 2019)

This quote is illustrative of someone who identifies as trans but who has lived with that identity being a secret and possibly someone who has not taken any steps towards transitioning. They describe a life where this has led to them feeling they have led a 'false life', which in turn has closed opportunities to develop a strong social network. For those who, for whatever reason, have begun their transition in later life or have had their transition interrupted by a terminal or life-limiting diagnosis, transition-related healthcare will continue to be an important part of their care at end of life. Recent research has highlighted that there may be barriers to these conversations continuing for many (Hospice UK, 2023).

While others may have good networks of support, it can still be difficult to think about who an individual might be able to call upon to care and advocate for them at the end of life. There is some evidence to suggest that trans individuals are also less likely than LGB people to engage in end-of-life planning such as will writing or appointing a healthcare proxy (Kcomt and Gorey, 2017). An additional issue to address is the full recognition of important relationships of care and support that may fall outside traditional conventions of heterosexual and cisgender relationships. For many trans and gender diverse people, their nominated 'next of kin' will not be a legal spouse or a blood relative. Westwood (2013) has questioned the extent to which contemporary law is adapting to take account of changing relationship forms, particularly with friendships becoming more significant in the lives of many, especially in later life and with reference to recognition of LGBT carers within key UK socio-legal policy discourses. There is a potential danger of some support networks being excluded in a number of ways, for example not being able to have an active role in the care of the dying or by not having their grief acknowledged (Walter, 1999). These issues are also important to consider in the drafting of wills to ensure that the testator's wishes are met.[1]

Concerns have been identified by trans people relating to what happens after they die (Bristowe et al, 2018; Almack, 2019; Whitestone et al, 2020), in particular questions as to whether their family members would honour their wishes to have their gender accurately reflected on their death certificate and gravestone:

'On my demise, my daughters, I'm absolutely sure, would insist that I get buried as their dad, and that shouldn't be allowed, that I feel pretty strongly about.' (Shirley, 70, trans woman; from the 'Last outing' study, Almack, 2019)

'I worry about being misgendered in death & about the queerness of my life being masked in order to meet a heteronormative standard of expectations around what death & funerals should be like'(Community survey respondent; 'I just want to be me' report, Hospice UK, 2023)

The Hospice UK report (2023) reports that often, for trans and gender diverse people, their motivations for making plans or preparations, and considerations about the end of life, were different from the general cisgender population or factored in additional concerns. In particular, survey respondents noted that they have actually made plans/put extra measures in place in the hope it will prevent unsupportive family members having any kind of control over funeral arrangements. For many, the particular worry is the impact that being memorialised under the wrong name and identity would have on their grieving partners/spouses and close friends.

The Gender Recognition Act 2004 states that a person should be legally regarded as their acquired gender in all aspects of life and death. Shirley had also applied for a Gender Recognition Certificate. Despite these protections, however, she was still not confident that this would be respected on her death. The Trans Safety Network notes that it is possible to record a different sex on a person's death certificate from that recorded on a birth certificate if the evidence shows on the balance of probabilities that that is how the deceased was known; it does not require a deed poll evidencing a change of name or a Gender Recognition Certificate.[2]

Conclusion and directions for future research

As described by a trans woman, even if trans people aren't being pathologised, they are still frequently being defined by pain and challenges, and it is important to recognise the joy:

> I believe it's those moments of joy that define us – the glimmers of gender euphoria that keep us taking our pills, growing our hair, fighting insurance companies for care, and trying to make space for every shade of the gender rainbow in our world. It's joy that will see us through. (Black, 2020)

Hospice UK's report (2023) observes that it is important to remember that there are many positive aspects to growing older as a trans person, which may continue to the end of life. This perspective should be kept in mind in future research.

To date, evidence that is available about trans end-of-life care is largely based on small qualitative samples. These studies provide an accumulative body of research, but larger studies are still to be developed. Furthermore, participants are often White, and more research is needed to explore intersections between race, ethnicity and ageing and to be inclusive of non-binary participants.

Box 12.1: Useful resources

- 'Transgender and non-binary people and cancer', Available from: https://outpatients.org.uk/trans-and-nonbinary/
- '"I just want to be me": trans and gender diverse communities access to and experiences of palliative and end of life care', Available from: https://www.hospiceuk.org/publications-and-resources/i-just-want-be-me
- 'Inclusive care of trans and non-binary patients' (British Medical Association), Available from: https://www.bma.org.uk/advice-and-support/equality-and-diversity-guidance/lgbtplus-equality-in-medicine/inclusive-care-of-trans-and-non-binary-patients
- 'Providing LGBT+ inclusive palliative and end-of-life care: recommendations for people working in health and social care organisations' (developed by the European Association for Palliative Care Task Force on Palliative Care for LGBT+ People), Available from: https://eapcnet.eu/eapc-groups/task-forces/improving-palliative-and-end-of-life-care-for-lgbt-people/
- 'Provider pack breaking down barriers to LGBTIQ+ inclusive cancer care', Available from: https://secureservercdn.net/160.153.138.201/04v.b4d.myftpupload.com/wp-content/uploads/2021/08/ProviderPackV1.pdf
- 'Hiding who I am: the reality of end-of-life care for LGBT people', Available from: https://www.mariecurie.org.uk/globalassets/media/documents/policy/policy-publications/hiding-who-i-am-the-reality-of-end-of-life-care-for-lgbt-people.pdf
- 'Being accepted being me: understanding the end-of-life care needs for older LGBT people', Available from: https://derbyshire.eolcare.uk/content/documents/uploads/toolkit-docs/Being-Accepted-Being-Me.pdf

---

Notes

[1] 'Will drafting considerations for transgender and non-binary beneficiaries', 30 June 2021, Available from: https://www.willwriters.com/blog/will-drafting-considerations-for-transgender-and-non-binary-beneficiaries/

[2] J. O'Thomson, 'Coroner confirms that GRC is unnecessary for correct name and gender on trans death certificates', Trans Safety Network, 23 April 2023, Available from: https://transsafety.network/posts/coroner-confirms-grc-death-cert/

References

Almack, K. (2019) '"I didn't come out to go back in the closet": ageing and end of life care for older LGBT people', in A. King, K. Almack, T.-Y. Suen and S. Westwood (eds) *Older Lesbian, Gay, Bisexual and Trans People: Minding the Knowledge Gaps*, London: Routledge, pp 158–71.

Almack, K. and King, A. (2019) 'Lesbian, gay, bisexual, and trans aging in a U.K. context: critical observations of recent research literature', *International Journal of Aging and Human Development*, 89(1): 93–107.

Almack, K. Seymour, J. and Bellamy, G. (2010) 'Exploring the impact of sexual orientation on experiences and concerns about end-of-life care for lesbian, gay and bisexual elders', *Sociology*, 44(5): 908–24.

Black, R. (2020) 'The joy of being trans', *Medium*, 20 October 2020. Available from: https://aninjusticemag.com/the-joy-of-being-trans-13e30c019981

Bristowe, K., Hodson, M., Wee, B., Almack, K., Johnson, K., Daveson, B.A. et al (2018) 'Recommendations to reduce inequalities for LGBT people facing advanced illness: ACCESSCare national qualitative interview study', *Palliative Medicine*, 32(1): 23–35.

Carpenter, C.S., Eppink, S.T. and Gonzales, G. (2020) 'Transgender status, gender identity, and socioeconomic outcomes in the United States', *ILR Review*, 73(3): 573–99.

Cartwright, C., Hughes, M. and Lienert, T. (2012) 'End-of-life care for gay, lesbian, bisexual and transgender people', *Culture, Health & Sexuality*, 14(5): 537–48. DOI: 10.1080/13691058.2012.673639

Catlett, L., Acquaviva, K.D., Campbell, L., Ducar, D., Page, E.H., Patton, J. et al (2023) 'End-of-life care for transgender older adults', *Global Qualitative Nursing Research*, 10. online first, March, Available from: https://journals.sagepub.com/doi/10.1177/23333936231161128

Fredriksen-Goldsen, K.I., Cook-Daniels, L., Kim, H.J., Erosheva, E.A., Emlet, C.A. Hoy-Ellis, C.P. et al (2014) 'Physical and mental health of transgender older adults: an at-risk and underserved population', *The Gerontologist*, 54(3): 488–500.

Gott, M., Morgan, T. and Williams, L. (2020) 'Gender and palliative care: a call to arms', *Palliative Care and Social Practice*, 14.

Harding, R. Epiphaniou, E. and Chidgey-Clark, J. (2012) 'Needs, experiences, and preferences of sexual minorities for end-of-life care and palliative care: a systematic review', *Journal of Palliative Medicine*, 15(5): 602–11.

Hospice UK (2023) '"I just want to be me": trans and gender diverse communities access to and experiences of palliative and end of life care', London: Hospice UK.

Kcomt, L. and Gorey, K.M. (2017) 'End-of-life preparations among lesbian, gay, bisexual, and transgender people: integrative review of prevalent behaviors', *Journal of Social Work End of Life and Palliative Care*, 13(4): 284–301.

Kneale, D., Henley, J., Thomas, J. and French, R. (2021) 'Inequalities in older LGBT people's health and care needs in the United Kingdom: a systematic scoping review', *Ageing & Society*, 41(3): 493–515.

Koffman, J., Bajwah, S., Davies, J.M. and Hussain, J.A. (2023) 'Researching minoritised communities in palliative care: an agenda for change', *Palliative Medicine*, 37(4): 530–42.

Lawton, A., White, J. and Fromme, E.K. (2013) 'End-of-life and advance care planning considerations for lesbian, gay, bisexual, and transgender patients', *Journal of Palliative Medicine*, 17(1): 106–8.

National Palliative and End of Life Care Partnership (2021) 'Ambitions for palliative and end of life care: a national framework for local action 2021–2026', Available from: https://www.england.nhs.uk/wp-content/uploads/2022/02/ambitions-for-palliative-and-end-of-life-care-2nd-edition.pdf

Pang, C., Gutman, G. and de Vries, B. (2019) 'Later life care planning and concerns of transgender older adults in Canada', *The International Journal of Aging and Human Development*, 89(1): 39–56.

Reisner, S.L., Poteat, T., Keatley, J., Cabral, M., Mothopeng, T., Dunham, E. et al (2016) 'Global health burden and needs of transgender populations: a review', *The Lancet*, 388(10042): 412–36.

Rosa, W.E., Roberts, K.E., Braybrook, D., Harding, R., Godwin, K., Mahoney, C. et al (2023) 'Palliative and end-of-life care needs, experiences, and preferences of LGBTQ+ individuals with serious illness: a systematic mixed-methods review', *Palliative Medicine*, 37(4): 460–74.

Rowley, J., Richards, N., Carduff, E. and Gott, M. (2021) 'The impact of poverty and deprivation at the end of life: a critical review', *Palliative Care and Social Practice*, 15.

Stinchcombe, A., Smallbone, J., Wilson, K. and Kortes-Miller, K. (2017) 'Healthcare and end-of-life needs of lesbian, gay, bisexual, and transgender (LGBT) older adults: a scoping review', *Geriatrics*, 2(1), Available from: https://doi.org/10.3390/geriatrics2010013

Walter, T. (1999) *On Bereavement: The Culture of Grief*, Buckingham: Open University Press.

Westwood, S. (2013) '"My friends are my family": an argument about the limitations of contemporary law's recognition of relationships in later life', *Journal of Social Welfare and Family Law*, 35(3): 347–63.

Whitestone, S.B., Giles, H. and Linz, D. (2020) 'Overcoming ungrievability: transgender expectations for identity after death', *Sociological Inquiry*, 90(2): 316–38.

Willis, P., Raithby, M., Dobbs, C., Evans, E. and Bishop, J.A. (2021). '"I'm going to live my life for me": trans ageing, care, and older trans and gender non-conforming adults' expectations of and concerns for later life', *Ageing & Society*, 41(12): 2792–813.

Witten, T.M. (2014) 'End of life, chronic illness, and trans-identities', *Journal of Social Work in End-of-Life and Palliative Care*, 10(1): 34–58.

Witten, T.M. (2016) 'The intersectional challenges of aging and of being a gender nonconforming adult', *Generations*, 40(2): 63–70.

Over to you

This section provides three suggested learning activities for readers that connect explicitly with the content and themes that have arisen in the final three chapters in Part III. These focus on the application of your learning to direct care practices that make a difference to improving care and support for trans people in later life.

Practitioners can use these learning activities to help develop and share knowledge, skills and values that will inform the development of affirmative and person-centred support for older trans people by:

- extending your own personal and professional knowledge through relevant desktop research or practitioner enquiry;
- facilitating critical reflection and learning through active discussion in your team and service.

Educators and trainers can use these activities to:

- include trans ageing issues in the education and training of the workforce;
- guide the aim and focus of trans issues, drawing on the relevant evidence provided.

Managers can use these activities to:

- embed the relevant topics, areas and learning resources into the recruitment, induction, supervision, appraisal and staff career progression process;
- keep a record of key activities that can be drawn upon in practice reviews or benchmarks to demonstrate how the needs of older trans people are being addressed including the potential to demonstrate legal compliance during statutory regulatory activities.

Activity 6: Supporting Amena

Case studies are designed to enable a more detailed and important understanding of issues that trans older people may face while there are gaps in the literature or in your direct experience. They draw on the book contributors' discussion of issues that may inform how practitioners can improve their practice. We have provided an outline of an individual story with some suggested questions to support individual reflection and/or active team discussion,

Amena's story

Amena is a trans woman of mixed heritage. Her father came to the UK from India after fighting with the Allies in the Second World War and married her English mother soon after. Amena was born in 1948 and is now in her 70s. She married Asfara at aged 26 and they had four children, and she reflects that this was on the whole a happy and supportive marriage. After retiring from a long career in the civil service, Amena decided to transition and began living as a woman in all aspects of her day-to-day life. She has been supported by a local community organisation who have helped her access some private services such as voice therapy and electrolysis. Amena continues to visit her local temple, where she perceives herself to be fairly anonymous and enjoys the spiritual support. Her wife had been supportive but in the last two years decided to move away to start her own new life. Since then, two of Amena's sons have been very aggressive towards her and have raised vociferous objections to Amena taking any further steps in her gender affirmation and have threatened to cut her off if she expresses her gender in public places. Their teenage grandchildren have also said that they don't want to visit Amena and at the last encounter called her a 'freak'. As they live locally, this is a very difficult situation, culminating in the family outing Amena to members of her local temple. As a result, Amena received some offensive and hurtful letters and phone calls from people she had known for a very long time as well as some supportive messages and offers to visit her at home.

To complicate matters, Amena recently had a small stroke which has impacted on her sight and to some extent her ability to travel locally with confidence. Amena feels that this threat to her independence has made her more visible, and whereas normally she would approach her temple for support, she now feels very vulnerable and isolated. She recently hired a local cleaner to give her some help with cleaning and meal preparation at home. In the last few days, however, she presented to her GP following a fall at home and on examination was observed to have some suspect fingertip bruising on her arms and a small burn on her back.

Questions for discussion and reflection:

1. What concerns might you or other members of your team have about Amena's presentation, and what would be the first steps to take to ensure her immediate wellbeing?

2. What might be some of Amena's concerns regarding arrangements for her current and future care, and what barriers might deter her from seeking support?
3. What support might Amena benefit from accessing, and what advice might she need?
4. How might different aspects of Amena's identity (ethnicity, gender, religion, family roles and age) intersect to affect her experiences and needs?
5. Are there any strengths or resiliencies in her life that you could help Amena to draw on?

Activity 7: Mapping resources and identifying networks to develop affirmative relationships with trans advocacy organisations

Taking purposeful action to improve the practice environment involves a planned and structured approach to learning and knowledge exchange between the community, professionals, practitioners and their organisations. The following suggestions for teams and individuals aim to help identify good practice, generate tailored and co-produced support and resources and come up with recommendations on how to make a difference through trans-affirmative practice. Use these to inform service development plans over time:

- Investigate the presence of local trans or LGBTQ+ groups in your local area, look at any websites and make direct contact either virtually or in person to share your interest in how your organisation can raise and demonstrate awareness of the trans community and their needs.
- Invite consultation on how your service can be more trans affirmative and inclusive of trans needs in later life. Make sure that you offer remuneration for any consultancy provided.
- Show support by offering to share resources, for example by making a meeting space available or assisting with advertising a group or network in your service literature or link to them online or provide a safe space in which trans groups can meet with service providers.
- Consider providing a named person whom advocates can contact to discuss any issues on behalf of individuals or the community.
- Develop a survey or consultation in partnership with a local trans or LGBTQ+ organisation.
- Show up at trans events locally or host an event in the trans cultural calendar.
- Always follow up and communicate any trans-affirmative developments in your service and find a way of getting feedback to stimulate ongoing relationships.
- Discuss how best to capture feedback on incidents of discrimination and transphobia that can be used to inform service improvement at both an individual and system level.

Activity 8: Developing a zero-tolerance statement on transphobia at your place of work

This task encourages you to discuss and develop a position statement and can be used to help convey a safe and supportive environment for people that should be based on a culture in which everyone is valued. A zero-tolerance attitude is one tool that can be developed and signed up to in order to demonstrate this environment.

To promote and uphold a zero-tolerance attitude towards transphobia in the workplace, you may wish to consider and address the following:

- how transphobic behaviours including misgendering will be challenged;
- how incidents will be reported and monitored;
- how trans and non-binary staff and people using services will be consulted and supported when discrimination occurs;
- how staff and people involved in the service will be trained as bystanders;
- the use of inclusive language in your statement so that it is as clear and understandable as possible and factually accurate;
- how the organisation/service/team is going to respond to any backlash.

★★★

This final section provides a suggested learning activity for readers that connects explicitly with the content and themes across all chapters. This final activity is all about applying what you have learnt from reading this book and engaging with the other learning activities. The key focus is on promoting the autonomy, preferences and wishes of the older person – taking a person-led approach to trans-inclusive, affirmative care.

Practitioners can use this activity to help develop and share knowledge, skills and values that will inform the development of affirmative and inclusive support for older trans people by:

- reflecting on your professional responses to a practice-based scenario and considering how you would respond and what good support would look like;
- facilitating critical reflection and learning through active discussion among your team and service.

Educators and trainers can use this activity to:

- include trans ageing and care issues in the education and training of the workforce;
- facilitate discussions that are practice-near and invite participants to apply their learning from the book to a practice-based scenario.

Managers and leaders can use this activity to:

- embed the application of skills, knowledge and values into recruitment, induction, supervision, appraisal and career progression processes;
- assess pre-existing and current staff members' knowledge, awareness and ethical orientation towards supporting older trans people in a practice-based approach.

We have provided a further scenario which you can consider and discuss either individually or as part of a learning group.

Think about your responses to the scenario and questions and the messages and themes across this book.

Eric's story (he/they)

Eric (pronouns he/they) is an 81-year-old White trans man who has recently moved into a care home in his local area. Eric has lived in the local area for 40 years and used to be a well-known electrician and decorator in the area who ran his own business during the last decade of his working life. Eric had two long-term relationships during his earlier years – his most recent partner (his wife) died from liver cancer ten years ago, and Eric has lived alone since. Eric does not have any children and very little contact with extended family, except for Eric's brother and sister who also live in the local area. Eric has chronic obstructive pulmonary disease and experiences difficulty breathing, has a chronic cough and often feels tired. This limits his mobility and level of movement, and he rarely leaves the nursing home but does enjoy time in the surrounding gardens and visiting the park next to the nursing home when accompanied by a carer or one of his siblings. Eric used to attend the trans pride events held every year in the neighbouring city but finds it too exhausting to travel and attend now. Eric is also showing early signs of cognitive decline: he sometimes forgets how to get back to his room or gets lost in the home, does not always recognise staff members and needs daily assistance and reminders on what medications to take (including testosterone gel) and when to use his inhaler.

More recently, Eric has begun to describe himself as 'she' on some days, and at his request his sister has brought in some colourful blouses that he finds comfortable to wear. Eric's brother and his wife having Lasting Power of Attorney for Eric. They are in conflict with Eric's sister and her partner, and they have recently attempted to stop Eric's sister from visiting him. They have argued to the home manager that Eric's sister is not acting in his best interests and is confusing him and other residents by bringing in women's clothes. Eric's brother visits nearly every day and sometimes prevents care workers from entering Eric's room, claiming he is providing care for Eric that day and no one else needs to see him.

Eric's sister has also been in touch with the home manager to express her concerns about the controlling behaviour of their brother over Eric and that in the past Eric's brother has struggled to accept Eric's gender and frequently misgenders him, especially when talking about Eric to other family members. Eric's sister is also worried that their brother has tried to stop two of Eric's friends from visiting him in the home – two trans women who have been friends with Eric for many decades. This week, the home manager has received a report that a new member of care staff in the home has refused to provide support to Eric with bathing and dressing, stating that his body is "ungodly", he is not a "real man" and "not how God intended". Another care worker has noticed some bruises on Eric's upper left arm; Eric states he fell out of bed and does not want to talk about it.

Summary learning points

- What is your initial response to this scenario? What are the key concerns for Eric? What might be impacting his wellbeing? Consider his social, emotional, psychological and physical wellbeing and his rights and safety.
- How would you promote Eric's autonomy? Who else would you need to speak to?
- What support might Eric need in the short and medium term? What services might be beneficial to him?
- What would **inclusive and trans affirmative support** look like for Eric? What principles and values would you follow? What would you need to know more about and who might you consult?
- Share and discuss your responses with other colleagues in your service or with a manager or service lead in a supervision session.

Conclusion: Looking ahead for enabling trans-inclusive and affirming practice

Paul Willis, Michael Toze and Trish Hafford-Letchfield

The big messages

In this final chapter, we revisit the 'big takeaway messages' for health, community and social care practitioners that are woven across the chapters in this book, and we identify some future directions in research for supporting trans people in later life and developing trans-inclusive research and practice. In relation to improving care experiences across health and social care systems, a resounding message is the importance of developing and delivering a person-centred, person-led approach to care that is collaborative and centred on the wishes and preferences of older trans people as the experts on their lives. Promoting the autonomy of older trans people is an underpinning principle for delivering trans-inclusive and affirming practice.

Numerous authors in this book have stressed the importance of adopting an intersectional lens for better understanding older trans people's lives and the heterogeneity among this population. We would add to this the diversity between *different generations* of older trans people, as noted in Heyam's chapter (Chapter 10) on trans histories. Experiences of earlier life points will vary according to different generational cohorts in parallel with the chronological points when trans individuals 'come out' as trans. An intersectional lens deepens understanding of the complex connections between ageism and cisgenderism, and how these points of social marginalisation can undermine positive ageing experiences for trans people. The importance of recognising and assessing the social support networks of older trans people is another critical theme, taking into account the complexity of relationships with family members over time, potential experiences of familial estrangement and the scope of 'families of choice' for providing support in later life. A final resounding message is the ethical responsibility of helping professionals, such as social workers, community workers and healthcare professionals, to advocate for older trans individuals and to ensure that services for and accessed by older people are trans inclusive, cisnormative-critical and safe to access. As noted by Castle and Kimberley in their chapter, affirming experiences accessing healthcare will then lead to individuals feeling more willing to seek out healthcare services and clinicians.

Developing trans-inclusive research and scholarship – looking forward

In their chapter, Kneale et al highlight several takeaway messages for future research in this field (Chapter 1). An overarching message is the identified disparity between theories on trans ageing and the severely lacking availability of empirical evidence to support this. Kneale et al stipulate a note of caution to avoid adopting a deficit-only lens for understanding trans individual's wellbeing and relationships. We support this. Inevitably, a book that is primarily focused on the care and support needs of older trans people leans more towards a deficit agenda, that is, what goes wrong in the care of older trans people and how this can be remedied. Accordingly, one key area for future research is developing a richer understanding of older trans individuals' resiliency in overcoming often adverse, cisnormative arrangements and circumstances in their current lives and at earlier life points. What is needed is a stronger focus on how older trans people experience 'queer joy' in their everyday lives and how this contributes to their wellbeing. 'Queer joy' is discussed as an affective positive state and a point of resistance to heteronormative, cisnormative arrangements that recognises queer-affirming life experiences beyond more problem-saturated stories of queer (including trans) people's lives as dominated by accounts of distress and trauma (see Copeland, 2023 for a more detailed discussion). A fundamental question is how applicable this notion is to older people's wellbeing and how trans people in later life exercise this through their relationships with others. Through a generational comparative approach, what might be learnt about the ways in which younger and older trans people experience and exercise queer joy and everyday pleasure? And how might this learning be shared across generations? Linked to this is the significance of recognising positive experiences of growing older as a trans person, as touched upon in Almack et al's chapter (Chapter 12). This is essential when considering that many trans people may transition and seek to access gender-affirming treatments in later life; older age becomes a critical time of affirming change and self-actualisation.

Connected to the idea of joy is the importance of sexual pleasure. There is increasing attention on aspects of sexual wellbeing for older people belonging to sexual minority groups, mainly lesbians and gay men, but much less attention is given to the sexual rights and intimate relationships of older trans people (Simpson et al, 2023; one exception being Scarrone Bonhomme, 2022). The intersections between sexual health and sexual relationships, older age, gender transitioning and gender non-conformity warrant further research. This is in parallel with a greater focus on the romantic relationships of older trans people and how these potentially bolster the resilience and quality of life of trans individuals in later life. Integral to a focus on care and support in later life is the need to recognise disabilities and ableism and how these social dimensions intersect with, and potentially compromise, older people's wellbeing. Some authors in this book have touched on the impact of dementia, cognitive impairments and physical disabilities (see Chapters 7 and 11). However, more work is needed on understanding the wishes and expectations of trans disabled people for current and future care arrangements and, through a critical gerontology lens, how social disadvantage can accumulate across the life course and compound social and economic disparities in older age for trans disabled people.

A final area to highlight for more research is older trans people's use of and reliance on digital technology. We know from previous work that the arrival of the internet in the 1990s brought with it much-needed access to trans personal accounts and online groups and communities that were not easily accessible before (see Willis et al, 2021). Trans lives, identities and stories became much more visible through the internet and subsequent Web 2.0 platforms. Has this equipped older trans people with greater skills in digital literacy compared to cisgender older people, and what contributions have digital technologies made to older trans people's social networks and supportive relationships? An additional question is how digital technology may improve older people's engagement with health and social care providers, especially for those experiencing high levels of social isolation, and the ways in which digital platforms may enhance pathways of care for those accessing gender-affirming treatments and transitioning through medical means (as noted in Castle and Kimberley's chapter, Chapter 8). As highlighted by authors in this book, it is critical to actively involve trans people in research design and the delivery of studies about their lives and experiences. Research involvement and participation should be an empowering and affirming experience that brings tangible benefits to trans groups and communities. In a similar vein, Hafford-Letchfield and McCormack (Chapter 9) reiterate the need for trans-positive, evidence-based models of practice grounded in the experiences of trans people in later life. Local research about trans experiences and care needs is just as critical for informing good service delivery as wider programmes of funded research in this area.

Developing trans inclusive practice – looking forward

In this final section, we return to the big messages for developing trans-inclusive practice with older people. The 'Over to you' learning activities located across this book are one useful base for developing your knowledge and skills as helping professionals and practitioners. The bulk of these activities reiterate the importance of critical reflection – reflecting on your past experiences of supporting trans people (whether this be positive or not so positive), reflecting on the cisnormative and ageist beliefs and views we are bombarded with from childhood onwards within contemporary social climates and reflecting on the ways we can develop and deliver anti-oppressive practice. In the context of this book, this means practice that is *anti-cisnormative, anti-ageist* and grounded in an *intersectional* lens on marginalisation and social disadvantage. Critical reflection requires reflecting individually and collectively on the power and authority helping professionals hold, and being open to recognising that the ways in which we exercise power in relationships with service users and patients can inadvertently reinforce heteronormative and cisnormative arrangements. For example, not attending to regular usage of binary language in conversations, in data collection and in recording, or not considering how older people accessing your service may have trans-related needs. To help develop this critical approach, we encourage readers to return to the learning activities, to embed trans-inclusive practices into everyday work with people in later life, to regularly engage in 'trans-inclusive talk' as a service team and with other professional colleagues and to use the resources and reading identified across the chapters in this book to keep extending your knowledge of this area.

This learning development relies on supportive work cultures that are enabled through good leadership. The current social and political climate in the UK (and other Global North nations) frequently legitimises anti-trans rhetoric. Within this hostile context, it is crucial that organisational leaders set out and commit to a clear agenda for delivering trans-inclusive culture and practices 'from the top' and lead by example. This also means supporting staff in their knowledge development about trans issues in later life, including trans histories, and developing the legal literacy that is needed to provide good support for trans people seeking to transition socially and/or medically. Health and social care professionals can be called upon to advocate for older trans people; this is even more fundamental for supporting individuals experiencing declines in cognition and living with dementia. As reiterated throughout this book, trans-inclusive practice rests on a shared value base of upholding the autonomy and dignity of older trans people, adopting a person-led approach and practising from an anti-ageist and anti-cisnormative value base.

Final activity: so what next?

After having read this book:

- What questions do you still have? Where might you seek out further information and guidance?

- Identify three things you will do differently (a) in your practice and (b) as a service to promote a **trans-inclusive, affirmative approach** to your work with older people. How will you know you have achieved these things? What will be different in your practice and in your service?
- Who else in your team/service may find it useful to read this book and engage with the learning activities?

References

Copeland, S. (2023) 'Sustaining queer joy and potentiality: through independent production with homoground music podcast', *Journal of Popular Music Studies*, 35(4): 111–24.

Scarrone Bonhomme, L. (2022) 'The age of rediscovery: what is it like to gender transition when you are 50 plus?', in T. Hafford-Letchfield, P. Simpson and P. Reynolds (eds) *Sex and Diversity in Later Life: Critical Perspectives*, Bristol: Policy Press, pp 163–80.

Simpson, P., Reynolds, P. and Hafford-Letchfield, T. (eds) (2023) *Desexualisation in Later Life: The Limits of Sex and Intimacy*, Bristol: Policy Press.

Willis, P., Raithby, M., Dobbs, C., Evans, E. and Bishop, J. (2021) '"I'm going to live my life for me": trans ageing, care, and older trans and gender non-conforming adults' expectations of and concerns for later life', *Ageing & Society*, 41(12): 2792–813.

Index

A

abuse, intimate and domestic 152–3
 barriers to accessing services 160–2
 barriers to help seeking 159–60
 domestic abuse recognition and identification 157–9
 epistemological, political and social context 155–7
 influencing and shaping practice 162–4
 structural barriers 162
 violence against trans people 153–5
acceptance 81
accessibility 108, 141, 142, 158
 see also surgery
acrimony 84
activism (activists) 63, 100, 183
activities 85, 97
advocacy 19, 162
ageing, after surgery 139
ageing and care, trans, current situation 1
 demographics 5–6
 gender diversity and life course 6–7
 practical issues 8–9
 terminology 2–5
ageing, research studies evidence 15–18, 33–4
 ageing and preparedness 32–3
 health services and barriers 31–2
 lives and trajectories 23–4
 mental health, social support and inequalities 30–1
 observation from datasets 20–3
 physical health and inequalities 29–30
 publication trends and study designs 24–9
 stigma and violence 32
 theoretically driven guidance 18–20
ageing, trans masculine 91–3, 100–3
 autoethnographic account 96–9
 COVID-19, wellbeing and body image 99–100
 introspective approach to current literature 95–6
 literature limitations 94–5
 trans gerontological literature 93–4
Ageing with Pride Study 28
ageism 135–7
agency 19, 69, 161
Ahmend, A. 191
Almack, Kathryn 8, 222
anatomical reconstruction 139–40
animals, companion 160
Ansara, Y.G. 2
anxieties 100, 109
assumptions 125, 126
austerity 34, 72
Australia 85, 108, 206
Authentic Equity Alliance (AEA) 156
authentic self 195, 199
autoethnography 102
autonomy 140–1
avoidance, healthcare 47

B

Baril, A. 195
Barker, M. 197
barriers 6, 31–2, 52, 135, 209
 to accessing services in DA 160–2
 ageing bodies 93
 to help seeking in DA 159–60
 professionals 107–8
 structural 162
Bartholomaeus, C. 111
Behavioural Risk Factor Surveillance System (BRFSS) 21, 28
Benjamin, Harry 182
Bentham, Jeremy 193
bias 34, 137
body image 99–100
Bornstein, D.R. 160
Bouman, W.P. 31, 68, 78
Brazil 154
British Journal of Psychiatry 186
Brown, N.T. 156
bullying 158

C

Caceres, B.A. 191
Callahan, Evelyn 8, 15, 67, 77
campaigning 69–72
Canada 206
care 69–72, 137
 see also health services
 care building and refusing *see* non-agreement
 care environments 158
 care facilities 143–4
 care, informal 81
 care services 161, 198
 care settings, dementia 193–6
Castle, Elijah R. 7, 221
Cauldwell, David O. 182
Census, UK 2021 22–3
Charlson comorbidity index 138
children 8, 50–1, 79–80, 84
cis (cisgender), definition 2
cisgenderism, definition 2

Index

cisnormative, definition 2
class, social 101
coercive queering 6
collaborations 138, 188
colonisation 6
coming out 83
communications 84, 199
communities 22, 184, 223
  practice perspectives 63, 69–72, 86, 141–2
Comprehensive personalised Care Model 205
compromise 84
confidence 130
  trans clients 111–12
conflicts 200
consent, informed 44, 109
consequences 84
conversion therapy 22, 49, 109
Cook-Daniels, L. 163
cost-of-living crisis 34
costs 69
counselling 83, 163
COVID-19 pandemic 16–17, 30, 34, 72, 85, 99–100
Cox, Laverne 65
Crenshaw, K. 192
criminalisation 4
culture 3
curriculum, trans-inclusive 116–17

D

dam bursting 51
DASH checklist 163–4
data 115, 134, 137, 139–40, 143, 153
data collection 5–6
datasets 20–3, 62, 81, 109
death 84, 114, 209–10
death, premature 62
dementia 41, 94–5, 114, 186, 200, 223–4
  see also neutrality, gender
demographics 5–6
depression 79
deprivation 206
determination, personal 69
diagnostic criteria 186–7
dialogues 93
digital literacy 141, 223
dignity 141
disability 97, 101, 154, 159, 163
discrimination 8
  abuse 159, 160–2
  ageing bodies 93
  families 79–80, 86
  inclusivity 192, 197, 206, 208
  professionals 108, 117
  refusing care 62
  research 19, 32, 46
  surgery 136
  Sweden 120

diseases, noncommunicable 32
disenfranchisement, societal 136
disparity 34
diversity 91, 208, 221
  gender 3
divorce 8
domestic abuse (DA)
  definition 153
  see also abuse, intimate and domestic
dysphoria 47, 101, 158

E

education 101, 142
Ellis, Carolyn 96, 102
embodiment 99
embodiment, gendered 135–7
encouragement 46
end-of-life care 204–5
  conclusion and future research 210–11
  research 205–10
energy levels 97
English Longitudinal Study of Ageing (ELSA) 16, 20
enhanced recovery after surgery (ERAS) protocol 138
Equalities Office LGBT survey 78
equality 127–8, 179
Equality Act (2010) 62, 114, 156
Equality and Human Rights Commission 156–7
equitable access *see* surgery
equity 91
estrangement, family 85
ethnic groups 30, 211
European Commission 120
exclusion 64, 161, 162, 206
exclusion, socioeconomic 8
expectations 43
experiences 61, 85
  conceptualising trans 183–4
  medical and social transition 184–5
  naming trans 182–3

F

Fabbre, Vanessa D. 42, 51, 63, 188
familiarity, trans people and issues 111–12
families 50, 77–8, 85–7, 198
  abuse 157, 162
  insights 81–4
  parenting 78–81
  surgery 142
fat deposits 97, 98
fears 94, 120, 159, 162, 195, 198
finances 206
financial privilege 101
FORGE project 162–3
Foucault, M. 193, 195, 199
fragmentation 71
frailty 138

227

Fredriksen-Goldsen, K.I. 19, 31
friends 85
funding 71, 72

G

gaps 34, 94, 108
  Trans Ageing and Care (TrAC) study 110–16
gaps, knowledge 33
gaslighting 158
gatekeeping 64, 96, 101
gender 52, 184
Gender Affirmation framework 20
gender diversity 62, 192
  life course 6–7
gender expression 194, 199
gender identities 5, 99, 108, 158, 197, 208
  families 78–9, 81, 85–6
  Sweden 121, 128, 131
  see also neutrality, gender
gender identity clinics (GICs) 43, 186
gender inversion 184
Gender Minority Stress Framework (GMSF) 18
gender-non-conformity 182
  see also neutrality, gender
Gender Recognition Act (2004) 113, 116, 210
Gender Recognition Certificate 113–14, 156, 210
generativity 86
Global North 3, 62
Global Social Work Statement of Ethical Principles 123
Global South 5
globalisation 6
Golub, S.A. 137
Government Equalities Office 21
grandchildren 83, 84
grandparents 78
groups 141, 159
Guadalupe-Diaz, X.L. 160
guidance 18–20
guidelines 116, 122, 127
gynecomastia 92

H

Hafford-Letchfield, Trish 9, 198, 223
hair removal 47–8
Harding, R. 206
Harper, Phil 8, 191, 196, 198
Harris, J.K. 29
hate crimes 162
health 6, 7, 20, 96, 120
Health and Retirement Survey 20
Health Equity Promotion Model 19
health outcomes 85
health services 31–2, 198
  experiences 66–9
healthcare 8, 87, 93, 96, 107–8, 134

healthcare navigation 41–2
  hair removal 47–8
  HRT 44–5
  screenings 45–7
  surgery 48
  transitioning later in life 48–52
  waiting times 42–4
healthcare providers 31
Henry, R.S. 33
Herman, J.L. 156
heteronormativity 193
Heyam, Kit 7
Hillman, J. 32, 154–5
Hirschfeld, Magnus 182
history, trans 179–80, 187–8
  changing terminology, concepts and experiences 180–5
  production of realness 185–7
homelessness 80, 159
homes 153
homicides 153
homogenisation 181
honesty 84
honour-based abuse 157
Hospice UK 210
hospitalisations 155
housing 143, 159
Howerton, I. 29
HRT 44–5
Human Dignity Trust 4

I

identities 19, 28, 49, 158–9, 186–8, 206
  ageing bodies 93, 95, 97
  gender neutrality 191–2, 196, 201
  see also gender identities
implants 140
inclusion 91
incomes 80, 160
independence 32, 140
inequalities 162, 205
  financial 141
inequities 159
information 49–50, 110–11, 163, 207–8
  surgery 134, 137, 142
information sharing 64
informed consent 44, 109
insecurities, professional 126–7, 130
insecurity 206
institutions 125, 136, 139, 140
Integrating care for Trans Adults (ICTA) project 41–2
internet 64, 223
intersectionality 163, 206, 211
  ageing bodies 93–5, 100, 102
  gender neutrality 191–2, 196
intersex 183–4, 186
interventions 163
interviews 41, 121–2, 124

intimate partner violence (IPV) 152
  definition 153
  see also abuse, intimate and domestic
intracommunity support 141–2
inversion 184
invisibility 116, 130, 152
Iridescent Life Course framework 19
isolation
  abuse 159
  ageing bodies 94
  end-of-life care 206, 208
  families 85
  refusing care 65
  surgery 140

J

Jordan, S.P. 161, 162

K

Kimberly, Laura L. 7, 221
Kitwood, T. 197
Klein, A. 137
Kneale, Dylan 222
knowledge 33
  families 86
  inclusivity 179, 193
  professionals 108–9, 117
  refusing care 69, 73
  surgery 137, 142
  Sweden 124–8, 130–1
  trans issues in later life 112–15
Koob, R.M. 196

L

language
  abuse 161
  ageing bodies 99
  gender neutrality 193, 196–7
  professionals 110
  Sweden 124, 126, 129
Lawler, S. 194
legal interventions 161
legal issues 117
legislation 87, 122, 127, 128
lesbian, gay, bisexual, transgender, queer and others (LGBTQ+) 15, 16–17, 19, 34, 61, 121
Lickert scale 111
life course theory 19
limitations 100
literacy, digital 141
literature 80, 155, 198, 205
  introspective approach 95–6
  limitations 94–5
  trans gerontological 93–4
lives and trajectories 23–4
loneliness 84, 85, 159, 160
long-term care 140–1
longevity 15

M

magazines 64
malignant social psychology (MSP) 197
marginalisation 5, 16, 208
  practices 63, 94, 102, 136
marriage 51
masculinity 92–3
mask wearing 100
McCormack, Keira 223
measures, validated 109
media 111, 116, 157, 186
medical treatments 95
menopause 44
mental health (illness) 62, 84, 94, 120, 155, 158
Messinger, A.M. 154
micro-aggressions 94, 96, 99, 163, 196–7
military service 30
minorities 17, 30
misgendering 91–2
Mollitt, P.C. 109
Morgan, Deborah 8
Morgan, L.M. 3
mortality 85

N

Nadal, K.L. 197
names 62
Nash, Adrienne 185
National Health Service (NHS) 45, 66–7, 68, 205
National Institute for Health research 41
National LGBT Survey 33
National Palliative and End of Life Care Partnership 204
National Surgical Quality Improvement Program (NSQIP) 138
navigation *see* non-agreement
negotiations 84
networks 64, 71, 72, 161, 208–9, 221
neutrality 187
neutrality, gender 190–1
  dementia care settings and power 193–6
  impact of incorrect terminology and language 197
  micro-aggressions and language 196–7
  professionals working 198–9
  recommendations 199–201
  translocational positionality, intersectionality and identity 191–2
Nokoff, N.J. 31
non-agreement 72–3
  experiences of community, campaigning and care 69–72
  experiences of formal health services 66–9
  transition pathways and possibilities 64–6
  vulnerability, robustness and resilience 62–4

writing about trans ageing 61–2
non-binary, definition 2
nursing homes 140, 144, 155

O

offence, causing 129
Office for National Statistics 22
online groups 223
online platforms 142
online spaces 64, 134, 141
oppression 16, 19, 136, 181
  ageing bodies 93, 95, 100
organisations 123, 130, 131
  non-profit 121
othering 141, 208

P

palliative care
  definition 204–5
  see also end-of-life care
Pang, C. 141, 208
parenting 78–81
  see also families
participants 22
partners 157, 198
partnerships 72
passing 154
Pearce, R. 7, 43, 64
peers 141, 159
pensions 114
persecution, state 62
police encounters 161
polycythaemia 69
poverty 80, 120, 206
power 193–6, 199, 201, 224
Power of Attorney 114
practical issues 8–9
practices, professional 179
precarity 71
prejudice 64, 79, 194
preparedness 32–3
  professional 124, 130
  see also Sweden
prisons 193
privacy 124, 156
professionalism 123, 130
professionals 4
  ageing bodies 93–4, 99–102
  families 80–1, 86
  gender neutrality 191, 198–200
  refusing care 72
  Sweden 122–3
  see also views and attitudes, professional
pronouns 4, 99, 158, 186, 200–1, 219
  Sweden 125, 129–30
protection 130
protection, legal 62
protocols 67
public records 156

public spaces 160
publication trends and study designs 24–9

Q

queer joy 222
questionnaires 109, 110, 127

R

realness, production of 185–7
recognition, legal 8
record keeping 52, 207
recovery 138
reflection 123
  critical 224
rejection 9, 86, 160
relationships 9, 63, 97, 180, 209
  abuse 152, 155, 159–60
  see also families
reporting 143
research 6, 8, 86
  abuse 155, 157, 163
  end-of-life care 205–10
  future, end-of-life care 210–11
  surgery 137, 143
  see also ageing, research studies evidence
resilience 19, 62–4, 69, 72, 86, 222
resistance 63, 129, 162
resources 122, 131, 160
  financial 86, 134
respect 158
retirement 8
Richards, C. 197
Riggs, D.W. 111
robustness 62–4
Rogers, M.M. 157, 161, 191
Royal College of General
  Practitioners 107, 115

S

safe spaces 131, 161, 200
safety 157
sample sizes 28
SaveLives 163
scholarship 188
Schultz, J.W. 159
screenings (screening services) 32, 45–7, 163
self-definition 181, 187
self-determination 99, 187
self-disclosure 187
self-esteem 160
self-medication 64, 68
self-realisation 66
self-reflexivity 131
self-regulation 193–4
self-reliance 160
self, sense of 158
separation 8
Serano, Julia 91
services 161

Index

settings 196, 200, 207
  social work 124–5
sexual wellbeing 222
sexuality 136, 184, 186, 197
shame 103, 157, 159
shelters 160
Silverman, M. 195
Smolle, Sofia 8
social care 87, 107–8
social inclusion 69
social media 116
social networks 84, 142
social policies 85
social services 93
Social Services Act (2001) 121
social stressors 18
social support 20, 31–2
  see also families
social work (workers) 87, 109
  Sweden 123–9
societies 81
spaces 156
stakeholder 81
standards 116
stealth imperative 183–4
stereotypes 64, 125, 135–6, 142, 161
stigmatisation 32
  abuse 152
  families 79–80
  gender neutrality 198
  professionals 117
  surgery 136–7
  Sweden 120
Stonewall 15
strategies, social work 127–9
stress 163
  minority 86
stress, minority 96
stressors 160
structures, societal 128
studies 78, 79, 130, 137, 161
study designs 24–9
substance abuse 155
suicide 80, 155
support 125, 127, 131, 183
support groups (networks) 64, 69–72, 73, 141, 144, 208–9
support systems 50
surgery 48, 67, 134–5, 142–4
  ageing bodies 92–3, 99–102
  community support 141–2
  gender-affirming surgery and long-term care 140–1
  gender-affirming surgery in older age 137–40
  gendered embodiment and ageism 135–7
surveillance 193
surveys 41, 78, 107, 110, 154, 156
  see also Trans Ageing and Care (TrAC) study

Sweden 109, 120
  context 121
  profession and professionalism 122–3
  social work 123–9
  the study 121–2
  what can we learn? 129–31

T

Tan, K.K.H. 18
Transgender Resilience Intervention Model 19
technologies 100, 223
  assistive 138–9
terminology 2–5, 182, 197
testimonies, personal 187
therapists 109
threats 158
Towle, E.B. 3
Toze, Michael 30, 77, 94, 97
training 137, 163, 181
training, professional 115–16, 117, 121
Trans Ageing and Care (TrAC) study *see* views and attitudes, professional
trans and gender non-binary (TGNB) 85
trans and gender non-conforming (TGNC) 85
trans, definition 2
trans men, definition 2
Trans MetLife Survey 28
Trans Murder Monitoring (TMM) project 153
Trans Safety Network 210
trans time 181
trans women, definition 2
transgender 182
Transgender Emergence Model 20
transitioning 43
  families 81, 83
  inclusivity 135, 186, 206, 208–9
  later in life 48–52
  refusing care 64–6
  social 4
translocational positionality, intersectionality and identity 191–2, 196
transsexual 182–3
transvestite 182–3
traumas 102, 155, 156, 163, 222
trust 121, 137, 161

U

UK Household Longitudinal Study (UKHLS) 21
uncertainty 68
underfunding 20
understanding 128, 130
Understanding Society 21
  see also UK Household Longitudinal Study (UKHLS)
unemployment 80, 160

United Kingdom (UK) 34
  abuse. *see* abuse, intimate and domestic
  end-of-life care 204, 206
  families 78, 85
  professionals 107
  refusing care 62, 66, 72
United States of America (US) 34, 62, 134
  abuse 154, 162–3
  inclusivity 184, 206

V

Vaccaro, A. 196
variables 17
  demographic 109
Velocci, Beans 185
Vicente, Marta V. 181
victimisation 32, 160
videoconferencing 100
views and attitudes, professional 107–8
  ascertaining gaps 110–16
  background to study 108–9
  survey design and respondents 109–10
  trans-inclusive curriculum 116–17
Vincent, B. 196
violence 32, 83, 94, 152
  in DA 153–5
violence, social 93

visibility 125, 160
volunteers (voluntary sector) 72, 81
vulnerability 80, 120, 138
  abuse 154–5, 159
  end-of-life care 206, 208
  refusing care 61, 62–4

W

waiting times 42–4
Walker, R.V. 31
wellbeing 6, 108, 121, 160
  ageing bodies 99–100
  families 80, 85
Welsh Gender Services 116
Westwood, S. 155, 209
White, Francis Ray 97, 98, 99
Willis, Paul 206, 208
Witten, T.M. 6, 32–3, 63–4, 198, 204, 206
work methods, social work 127–9
work pressures 51
workforce 200
World Health Organization (WHO) 136, 204
World Professional Association for Transgender Health 116
wound healing 138

www.ingramcontent.com/pod-product-compliance
Lightning Source LLC
Chambersburg PA
CBHW051537020426
42333CB00016B/1965